OSCEs for the Final FFICM

T0201658

OSCEs for the Final FFICM

Raj Nichani
is a Consultant in Anaesthesia and Intensive Care Medicine, Blackpool Teaching Hospitals NHS Foundation Trust, Blackpool, UK

Brendan McGrath
is a Consultant in Anaesthesia and Intensive Care Medicine, University Hospital South Manchester, and Honorary Senior Lecturer at University of Manchester, UK

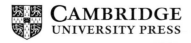

CAMBRIDGE
UNIVERSITY PRESS

University Printing House, Cambridge CB2 8BS, United Kingdom

One Liberty Plaza, 20th Floor, New York, NY 10006, USA

477 Williamstown Road, Port Melbourne, VIC 3207, Australia

314–321, 3rd Floor, Plot 3, Splendor Forum, Jasola District Centre, New Delhi –110025, India

79 Anson Road, 06–04/06, Singapore 079906

Cambridge University Press is part of the University of Cambridge.

It furthers the University's mission by disseminating knowledge in the pursuit of
education, learning and research at the highest international levels of excellence.

www.cambridge.org
Information on this title: www.cambridge.org/9781107579453

First published 2016
5th printing 2021

Printed in the United Kingdom by TJ Books Limited, Padstow Cornwall

A catalogue record for this publication is available from the British Library

Library of Congress Cataloguing in Publication data
Names: Nichani, Raj, author. | McGrath, Brendan, 1974- , author.
Title: OSCEs for the final FFICM / Raj Nichani, Brendan McGrath.
Description: Cambridge ; New York : Cambridge University Press, 2016. |
Includes bibliographical references and index.
Identifiers: LCCN 2016011814 | ISBN 9781107579453 (Paperback)
Subjects: | MESH: Critical Care | Great Britain | Examination Questions
Classification: LCC RC86.8 | NLM WX 18.2 | DDC 616.02/8–dc23 LC record available at
http://lccn.loc.gov/2016011814

ISBN 978-1-107-57945-3 Paperback

....

Every effort has been made in preparing this book to provide accurate and up-to-date information which is
in accord with accepted standards and practice at the time of publication. Although case histories are drawn
from actual cases, every effort has been made to disguise the identities of the individuals involved.
Nevertheless, the authors, editors and publishers can make no warranties that the information contained
herein is totally free from error, not least because clinical standards are constantly changing through
research and regulation. The authors, editors and publishers therefore disclaim all liability for direct or
consequential damages resulting from the use of material contained in this book. Readers are strongly
advised to pay careful attention to information provided by the manufacturer of any drugs or equipment
that they plan to use.

For Emma, Cerys and Bethan – thanks for the constant understanding and support and all the cups of coffee you brought down to the cellar whilst working on this book!

For Jaya, Neel and Taran – thank you for all your incredible encouragement, love and patience. Mum and Dad – for your untiring affection and strength of belief in me.

Contents

Section II: Equipment 177

Section III: Ethics and communication 221

Section IV: Resuscitation and simulation 251

Foreword

Intensive care medicine has become a speciality in its own right, bringing with it a new Faculty and examinations to become a Fellow of the Faculty of Intensive Care Medicine. A new examination needs new resources to help candidates prepare and revise and this book is aimed specifically at those preparing for the FICM OSCEs.

The authors have both had experience on both sides of the examining table and have been helping others through examinations since they completed their own training. The practice questions and model answers they have prepared are based on direct experience of the examination from recent candidates and represent accurately the type and range of questions one might expect. More importantly, the responses provided here are just what the examiners are looking for in answer to those questions.

This book will also have wider appeal to those wishing to broaden their knowledge of the sort of topics and situations that commonly arise in modern critical care practice. It is sure to also be invaluable to trainers and peers who are helping candidates prepare for these examinations and offer an insight into the complex and fascinating world of intensive care.

Peter Nightingale FRCA FRCP
Consultant in Anaesthesia & Intensive Care Medicine
Former Chairman of the Board of Examiners, Royal College of Anaesthetists
Intensive Care Unit
University Hospital South Manchester

Preface

The new Faculty of Intensive Care Medicine (FICM) comes with the inevitable faculty examinations and for the first waves of candidates, there were limited resources available to prepare from. For better or for worse, both of us have had plenty of experience of sitting examinations, both in intensive care medicine and other specialities. We both recognized the value of quality revision texts in focusing valuable revision time and in providing much needed exam-style questions to practice.

In our view, the ideal resource should reflect the examination question's style and content as much as possible, be a contemporary source of topical information and provide enough of an answer to save having to go and look something else up, saving time. This is what we have tried to achieve with this book and we hope you will find it extremely useful when preparing, revising or testing each other for the FICM OSCEs. We hope that it is also a valuable resource for anyone seeking to explore the curriculum of the FICM and gives an insight into the case mix, patients, technology and knowledge required to enjoy our speciality.

The questions are all matched to the syllabus domains and we have covered this as comprehensively as possible. The questions are largely based on candidate reports from recent exams. We have found the content both reliable and useful when preparing candidates over the last few years both informally and on our dedicated FICM examination revision courses. We thought it useful to incorporate an example marking scheme into the answers, we do however realize that we cannot replicate the examination marking scheme. In addition some questions have been left deliberately longer than what would be expected in a 7-minute examination, to allow us to cover as much relevant material as possible.

We would like to acknowledge the following people who have contributed to this book: Dr Andrew Bentley, Dr James Hanison, Dr Peter McDermott, Dr Daniel Nethercott, Dr Rob Thompson and Dr Anthony Wilson. We are grateful to the faculty of the North West FFICM Course for their help over the years and to candidates for their valuable feedback.

We hope that you will find the content useful. Good luck!

Raj & Brendan
Raj Nichani MB BS MRCP FRCA DICM FFICM
Consultant in Anaesthesia & Intensive Care Medicine
Blackpool Victoria Hospital

Brendan McGrath MB ChB MRCP FRCA EDIC DICM PGCertMedEd AHEA FFICM
Consultant in Anaesthesia & Intensive Care Medicine
University Hospital South Manchester

Disclaimer
Whilst every effort has been taken by the authors and publishers to ensure the accuracy of the information and data contained within this book, readers are advised to seek independent clarification and verification of the drugs, procedures and clinical guidance described in this book prior to undertaking clinical management. Neither the authors nor the publishers can accept responsibility for any injury or damage caused as a result of implementation of the work described in this book.

The FFICM – the examiner's view

FFICM Examiner

FFICM examiners observe a strict code of conduct, contributing to the integrity of the Faculty of Intensive Care Medicine and of the examination. Examiners cannot contribute questions to local or regional exam practice days. If they 'mock-examine' they may only use material provided by the local organizers. Examiners will attempt to observe a high level of information governance for question writing and standard setting. With this guidance in mind, this section is written by a current FFICM examiner in order to give an examiner's perspective of the exam itself and of what examiners are looking for in successful candidates. Specifically, Dr Clarke has not contributed to, reviewed, nor commented on the material contained within this book.

The FFICM in perspective

The FFICM is an integral part of both the standalone certificate of completion of training (CCT) in intensive care medicine, and the dual programme. Passing the examination is an entry requirement to speciality training level 7 (ST7) and as such the examination has been defined both by the General Medical Council (GMC), and previous examination chairs as a 'high stakes' examination – vital for both trainee career progression and for the protection of patients. The examination is both realistic and 'real world' with the Objective Structured Clinical Examination (OSCE) attempting to recreate a normal working day on a critical care unit. The success of this approach is evidenced by the visitor's comments after the March 2015 examination; the lay visitor's surprise at some candidate's failure to use antiseptic gel being especially telling. Underlying the more scientific and intellectual debates within our speciality is a constant focus on the simple basics of our practice.

The candidates

As parts of the old Diploma in Intensive Care Medicine were adapted to the current FFICM a problem for the examiners was that nobody knew what to expect of an ST6 on the new programme. Various definitions have arisen – usually around a trainee who could be expected to manage the unit overnight with remote supervision. The situation was complicated by the fact that many of the initial tranche of candidates were training on the old programme and were attempting the exam around the time of consultant interview. In early sittings the pass rate for the OSCE reached 100% emphasizing the high standard of early cohorts of candidates. The current view of examiners on standards can be summarized as:[1]

> a doctor in training who is familiar with the syllabus and has done the necessary bookwork. They would clinically be at the level of a registrar who would be able to formulate a plan of care for a critically ill patient with appropriate consultant backup.

It is not surprising that the standard of the examination evolves, which is important in quality assurance and standard setting.

Standard setting

As a 'high stakes' examination, standard setting becomes crucial. The FFICM examination has to fulfil the standards outlined in the GMC's 'standards for curricula and assessment', especially ST8 and ST12. Since 2014, the GMC has been able to access results at trainee level. A variety of tools are used in standard setting the examination – principally the Angoff, Ebel and the Hofstee scores.[2] The Angoff method is based on the concept of the borderline or minimally competent candidate whose knowledge, skills and attitude are just enough and who has a 50:50 chance of passing the examination. In other words, the borderline candidate is the marginal student: one whom on some days might just barely pass the examination but on other days might fail. It is important to note that this 'student' has done a reasonable amount of preparation for the theoretical examination. Importantly, this means the FFICM is *not* 'norm referenced'. In theory, 100% of candidates could pass (or fail). There is some evidence that examination pass rates are higher with the Angoff method than with norm-referencing.[3]

Angoff referencing is difficult for examiners and this bears on the debate around expectations of ICM trainees at the ST6 level. The essential point is that the FFICM is a fair examination. At the examiners 'call round' following the SOE and OSCE, debates have always been decided in favour of candidates, with the sole exception of ensuring that unfortunate precedents for the future are not set.

Examiners

The examiners are a mixed group. Although predominantly from teaching hospitals there are examiners from smaller units. Many will have held roles in training and education (often as regional advisers) and all have considerable experience in assessment. Some examine for other Royal colleges and have brought this experience to the FFICM. Specific examiners have been recruited as they have expert knowledge of standard setting, usually from involvement in medical school examinations.

You can't 'read' your examiner! They will invariably be pleasant and empathetic with you but this is no predictor of outcome. In the OSCE in particular, examiners must not prompt and you should not misinterpret a relatively flat affect as disengagement. There is an ongoing process of quality assurance and the floor supervisors, other examiners (on audit duty) and the visitors constantly assess and feed back on the examiner performance individually.

The MCQ

The multiple choice question (MCQ) is mapped to the curriculum domains and all questions are sampled to some extent. Single best answer (SBA) questions are now established and arguably are a better test of understanding as opposed to simple factual knowledge. The 'cover-up' test, whereby the stem and question are read and possible answers considered before looking at the available answers, is widely used by examiners in assessing new SBAs and can be invaluable to candidates in attempting the question. The pool of SBA questions is rapidly expanding, and unlike the multiple true false (MTF) questions, none are adapted from other colleges' question banks. The MTF questions are under constant review and redrafting in order to ensure they are fair and up to date. Unlike, say, the Royal College of Anaesthetists, the FFICM examiners have little historical data on the performance of MTF questions. At the standard setting meeting following each MCQ examination examiners have to justify the Angoff score they have given the question and it is this process that ultimately determines the pass mark.

The SOE

The Structural Oral Examination (SOE) seems to be the hardest part of the examination to pass – the pass rate in March 2015 being 62.3%. Candidates repeating the SOE, with a previous OSCE pass, struggle in particular, the pass mark for these candidates being 25%. There is some evidence from the initial sittings of the examination that the SOE is the most discriminating part of the examination.[4] The topics covered in the previous diet of the examination are listed on the FICM website, and really demonstrate how widely the curriculum is sampled. It really must be emphasized that in addition to 'state-of-the-art' research there is a concentration on the basics of clinical management and the day-to-day organization of a critical care unit. The March 2015 chairman's report comments on difficulties candidates had in describing the safe insertion of a nasogastric tube. Domain 11 of the curriculum deals with administration and management and Domain 12 deals with professionalism (and communication – invariably examined, usually in the OSCE). Attempts are made to map questions to all domains of the curriculum.

The OSCE

The OSCE can be intimidating, although traditionally candidates have done well in this part of the examination. There are stations on data interpretation, diagnosis and management, procedural skills, emergencies and communication. Simulation and actors are used. The OSCE is marked out of 20. It is perhaps the hardest part of the examination to examine as both candidates and the examiner are under pressure. There is additional pressure as the room can be noisy and the mannequin station especially can become intrusive. For the examiner, there is pressure to get the candidates through the entire question, such that marks at the end of the question can be scored.

Candidates should remember . . . !

- It's an OSCE – if you realize you have answered a question incorrectly you have not failed the OSCE. You have only lost 1–2 marks out of the 20. Keep moving forward and scoring the additional points.
- Should you remember an answer to a previous question after moving on, the examiner cannot go back and award marks. This is reasonable, as often subsequent questions will have given hints towards the answer, or even given a diagnosis.
- The examiner can't prompt, and indeed it is easy to foresee OSCEs being marked on tablet computers with only floor supervisors. If your examiner appears impassive they are only giving you adequate time to gain a mark.
- Equally, if your examiner cuts you short or moves you on, you should remember that their concentration is on ensuring you reach the available marks at the end of the station. There could be three marks available in the last 30 seconds. The examiner is acting in your best interests.
- There really are no killer stations and the eventual pass mark for the OSCE is determined by a standard setting process

There will be occasions where you have completed the OSCE with time remaining and either an uncomfortable silence will ensue or your examiner will engage in some small talk.

In preparing for the OSCE it is useful to remember that the chairman's report has constantly commented on candidate's relatively poor standards in data interpretation, especially ECGs. Continued data interpretation stations seem inevitable.

Good luck!

Dr Chris Clark

Consultant in Anaesthesia & Intensive Care Medicine, Blackpool Victoria Hospitals

References

1. Cohen AT. FFICM Examination – chairman's summary report. March, 2015

2. Holsgrove G. Reliability issues in the assessment of small cohorts. General Medical Council, Supplementary Guidance.

3. Mathysen DGP. Setting pass marks for examinations. CESMA meeting, Brussels, 28 November, 2009.

4. Webster N. FFICM Examination. *Critical Eye* 4: 15–17. 2013.

Introduction

Questions are included with expected answers. Each question has marks associated with it indicated in the [square brackets]. The total possible score for each OSCE question is 20 marks.

Many of the questions include tables of blood results. The following abbreviations are defined as follows:

APTT: activated partial thromboplastin time
BE: base excess
LDH: lactate dehydrogenase
INR: international normalized ratio
AST: aspartate aminotransferase
FiO_2: fraction of inspired oxygen
SpO_2: an estimate of arterial oxygen saturation
PO_2 (PCO_2): partial pressure of oxygen (carbon dioxide), which reflects the amount of oxygen gas (carbon dioxide) dissolved in the blood.

Other common abbreviations are: ECG, electrocardiogram; CT, computed tomography; MRI, magnetic resonance imaging; and HIV, human immunodeficiency virus.

Data 1

The medical registrar shows you some bloods from a patient who has a long-standing ileal conduit and presented with abdominal pain and vomiting to the surgeons.

		Reference range
Sodium	143 mmol/L	132–144 mmol/L
Potassium	4.4 mmol/L	3.5–5.5 mmol/L
Urea	9.8 mmol/L	3.5–7.4 mmol/L
Creatinine	162 µmol/L	62–106 µmol/L
Calcium	1.89 mmol/L	2.10–2.55 mmol/L
Corrected calcium	2.37 mmol/L	2.15–2.65 mmol/L
Glucose	5.1 mmol/L	4.0–5.9 mmol/L
Alkaline phosphatase	48 IU/L	40–129 IU/L
Albumin	16 g/L	34–48 g/L
Phosphate	1.69 mmol/L	0.7–1.4 mmol/L
Haemoglobin	7.2 g/dL	11.5–16.5 g/dL
Haematocrit	0.22	
FiO_2	0.21	
pH	7.3	7.35–7.45
pO_2	11.9 kPa	10.0–14 kPa
pCO_2	4.6 kPa	4.4–5.9 kPa
BE	−8.4 mEq/L	−2–+2 mEq/L
Lactate	2.9 mmol/L	0–2 mmol/L
Chloride	114 mmol/L	95–105 mmol/L
Bicarbonate	17.6 mmol/L	22–28 mmol/L

1. What do you make of these blood gases? What is the anion gap (AG)?

This is an example of metabolic acidosis. The chloride and lactate levels are elevated. [1]

You need to calculate the anion gap (AG), the principle of electroneutrality:

$$(Na^+ + K^+) - (Cl^- + HCO_3^-) \text{ is } (143 + 4.4) - (114 + 17.6) = 15.8 \text{ (normal AG acidosis).}$$

[1]

The normal value is 12–16 mEq/L – the difference is mainly due to the unmeasured negative charge on the proteins, sulphates and phosphates.

2. Is the albumin level significant?

Albumin is the major unmeasured anion and contributes almost the whole of the value of the AG. Low albumin will reduce the 'normal' gap. This should be commented on as it is relevant here. (Hypoproteinaemia is common in critical illness, albumin has a lot of negative charge.) A high AG acidosis in a patient with hypoalbuminaemia may appear as a normal AG acidosis if the low albumin is not corrected for. This albumin gap needs to be calculated as follows: [1]

The albumin gap $= 40 -$ apparent albumin

The AG corrected value $= $ AG $+$ (albumin gap$/4$).

It is generally accepted that the AG should be corrected upwards by 2.5 for every 10 g/L fall in the serum albumin. [1]

For this case, the albumin gap is $40 - 16 = 24$, making corrected AG $15.8 + (24/4) = 21.8$. This has changed an apparently normal AG acidosis into an increased AG acidosis.

3. Discuss the various causes of a normal and increased AG acidosis.

- Normal AG acidosis: [2 for most]
  - Disorders of bicarbonate homeostasis
  - Hyperchloraemia causes the acidosis
  - GI losses, vomiting, diarrhoea, renal losses, renal tubular acidosis, acetazolamide, iatrogenic (sodium chloride)
- Increased AG acidosis – increased 'unmeasured' anions: [2 for most]
  - Lactate, ketones, ethanol, asprin, cyanide, methanol, ethylene glycol
- Reduced AG acidosis – increased 'unmeasured' cations (for completeness):
  - Rare
  - Hypermagnesaemia, lithium toxicity, excess protein, myeloma
  - Waldenstrom's macroglobulinaemia (immunoglobulins are strong cations)

4. What is the cause of this acidosis in this patient? How would we clarify this?

This is a mixed picture. There is hypoalbuminaemia which complicates things.

You need to look for a cause of the raised AG, probably related to under-resuscitation, i.e. lactate, but it's worth checking ketones if there is prolonged starvation, and serum vs. calculated osmolarity if there is possible alcohol intoxication [2]

There is also hyperchloraemia. This may be iatrogenic following resuscitation but there will be an element of pre-existing derangement from the urinary diversion. [1]

5. How does the ileal conduit affect serum chloride?

The ileal conduit secretes bicarbonate into the lumen of the bowel in exchange for chloride. This results in bicarbonate loss from the body and excess chloride re-absorbtion. [2]

6. What is the strong ion difference (SID)? Explain.

The SID $= [Na^+] + [K^+] - [Cl^-]$; the normal value is 40 mmol/L. [1]

The pH, i.e. $[H^+]$, depends on the SID.

If you alter the value of SID, more or less water dissociates to maintain electroneutrality, hence altering $[H^+]$. Na^+ and K^+ are regulated strictly by other systems. The main 'metabolic regulator' is therefore Cl^-. [2]

In this case, SID $= 143 + 4.4 - 114 = 33.4$.

This would suggest that $(40 - 33.4 = 6.6)$ mmol/L of the base excess is attributable to the strong ion changes, namely a change in the Na:Cl ratio or hyperchloraemia.

7. What treatment would you suggest based on the arterial blood gases?

You need to ensure that tissue hypoperfusion is treated and corrected by seeing the base excess and lactate and urine output, etc. improve.

You may need to use flow haemodynamic monitoring to ensure good cardiac output in the face of hypotension.   [2]

8. Would you administer bicarbonate? What are the potential problems?

As a proportion of this problem is due to electrolyte problems, then correction of this may be justified in the form of bicarbonate. Ensure that any hypoperfusion is addressed first as this will just mask some of the 'perfusion markers'. Sodium bicarbonate necessitates a large sodium load and is said to cause a paradoxical intracellular acidosis through increased CO_2 generation.   [2]

Data 2

You are asked to review a 75-year-old patient in theatre recovery after a wide local excision and axillary node clearance for breast carcinoma. The patient was well pre-operatively, but started to become hypoxic during the 90-minute case. She was successfully extubated but her oxygen saturations are now reading at 85%. The rest of her observations are within normal limits.

1. **What is your approach?**

Check airway, breathing, circulation and give 15 litres oxygen via non-rebreathe bag. [1]

Take a history and carry out an examination. [1]

Check arterial blood gas. [1]

Order a chest X-ray. [1]

Aim to rule out causes such as airway compromise, hypoventilation, residual neuromuscular block, atelectasis and preumothorax. [1]

2. **This is her chest X-ray. What do you make of it?**

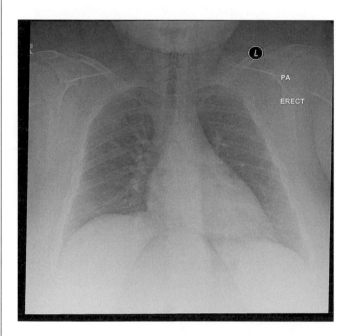

The heart is not enlarged. There is no lobar collapse, consolidation or gross pulmonary oedema. There is no pleural effusion. The major pulmonary vessels appear normal at the hilum. [1]

These are the results of a subsequent blood gas taken in theatre recovery on 60% FiO$_2$. Her oxygen saturations remain low at 85%.

		Reference range
FiO$_2$	0.60	
pH	7.38	7.35–7.45
pO$_2$	31.1 kPa	10.0–14 kPa
pCO$_2$	4.6 kPa	4.4–5.9 kPa
BE	−1.1 mEq/L	−2–(+2) mEq/L
Lactate	1.9 mmol/L	0–2 mmol/L

3. How would you calculate her alveolar–arterial (A–a) oxygen gradient? Why is it important?

This is calculated starting from the alveolar gas equation: [1]

$$PAO_2 = PiO_2 - PaCO_2/R$$

where

PAO$_2$ = partial pressure of oxygen in the alveoli

PiO$_2$ = partial pressure of inspired oxygen, which is = FiO$_2$ × (atmospheric pressure − water vapour pressure); atmospheric pressure = 101 kPa at sea level, water vapour pressure = 6.3 kPa

PaCO$_2$ = partial pressure of carbon dioxide in arterial blood

R = respiratory quotient = 0.8

The A–a oxygen gradient is calculated as follows:

$$A - a \text{ oxygen gradient} = PAO_2 - PaO_2$$

where

PaO$_2$ = partial pressure of oxygen in arterial blood

A high A–a gradient signifies an underlying problem with either a ventilation/perfusion (V/Q) mismatch or the presence of a shunt. The normal A–a gradient increases with age. [1]

4. Her A–a gradient is not unduly high. What do you think is wrong and what has caused this?

She has methaemoglobinaemia caused by the use of dye to help aid localization of lymph nodes. [2]

The low oxygen saturation is as a result of the absorption spectrum of methaemoglobin detected on pulse oximetry.

5. How would you confirm your diagnosis?

An arterial blood gas test using co-oximeter analysis shows elevated methaemoglobin levels.[2]

6. What are other known causes for this condition?

It can be congenital (cytochrome b5 reductase deficiency) or acquired. [1]

Acquired causes include exposure to drugs including: [1]

- Nitrates
- Certain local anaesthetics – e.g. prilocaine, benzocaine
- Certain antibiotics – e.g. dapsone
- Analine dyes

7. Explain the underlying pathophysiology.

The ferrous ion Fe^{+2} in haem is oxidized to the ferric state Fe^{+3}. Fe^{+3} ions have poor oxygen affinity. The remaining ferrous ions have increased oxygen affinity causing a left shift of the oxygen disassociation curve and reduced oxygen delivery to tissue.   [2]

8. What clinical features may you see?   [2 for all]

Symptoms are proportional to the fraction of methaemoglobin. A normal methaemoglobin fraction is about 1% (range, 0–3%). Symptoms associated with higher levels of methaemoglobin are as follows:

- 3–15% – Slight discolouration (e.g. pale, grey, blue) of the skin
- 15–20% – Cyanosis, though patients may be relatively asymptomatic
- 25–50% – Headache, dyspnoea, lightheadedness, weakness, confusion, palpitations, chest pain
- 50–70% – Abnormal cardiac rhythms; altered mental status, delirium, seizures, coma; profound acidosis
- > 70% – Usually, death

May be asymptomatic especially if levels < 15%.

9. What is the treatment for this?

Administer supplemental oxygen.   [1]

Intravenous methylene blue is a specific antidote, facilitating the reduction of methaemo- globin.   [1]

The role for hyperbaric oxygen and exchange transfusion remains anecdotal.

10. What other dyshaemoglobinaemias can cause spurious results with pulse oximetry?

Examples of other dyshaemoglobinaemias that can cause spurious results are carboxyhaemo- globin and sulfhaemoglobin.   [1]

Data 3

A 45-year-old man is admitted to the intensive care unit with fevers, tachycardia, abdominal pain and distension and profuse watery diarrhoea. He has a history of type I diabetes mellitus and received a cadaveric renal transplant 3 years ago for diabetic nephropathy. The following blood tests are obtained:

		Reference range
Sodium	147 mmol/L	136–145
Potassium	5.3 mmol/L	3.6–5.2
Urea	18 mmol/L	2.5–6.4
Creatinine	231 μmol/L	80–132
WCC	21.5×10^9/L	4–11
Neutrophils	20.3×10^9/L	2–7.5
Haemoglobin	10.1 g/dL	11.5–16.5
Platelets	467×10^9/L	150–400
Albumin	26 g/L	35–50
Total bilirubin	6 umol/L	3–17
ALT	47 IU/L	30–65
Alkaline phosphatase	63 IU/L	50–136

1. Describe the following radiograph.

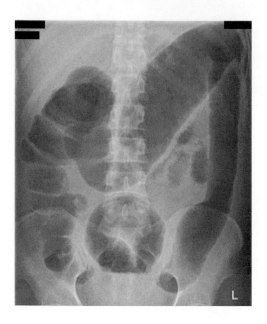

The plain abdominal film shows dilatation of the large bowel without obvious obstruction. There is evidence of bowel wall oedema with 'thumb-printing', and pseudopolyps or 'mucosal islands'.   [2]

2. What are the possible causes of his clinical presentation?   [3 for all]
This patient presents with toxic megacolon (systemic toxicity with a dilated, inflamed colon). The causes are:
- Infective causes:
  - *Clostridium difficile* infection
  - Cytomegalovirus colitis (in immunosuppressed patients)
  - Salmonella/shigella/campylobacter infection
- Inflammatory bowel disease (e.g. ulcerative colitis)
- Intra-luminal obstruction (e.g. tumour) with perforation and peritonitis (less likely in the context of diarrhoea)

3. What further diagnostic tests could be helpful?   [3 for all]
Send stool for culture.
Perform a CT scan of the abdomen. (Appearances may help to determine the cause of the dilatation whilst also excluding an obstructive cause. In addition it may detect complications such as perforation or vascular compromise.)
You might consider *cautious* flexible sigmoidoscopy. A colonoscopy is not recommended due to the risk of perforation.

4. How can you classify diarrhoea? [4 for all]

It can occur as a consequence of four different mechanisms:

1. Osmotic: excess osmotically active solutes in the gut lumen, which retain water. Examples include magnesium salts, bile salts (malabsorption) and some laxatives (e.g. lactulose – a synthetic, non-digestible sugar).
2. Secretory: often caused by enterotoxins from *Vibrio cholerae* or *E. coli*.
3. Inflammatory: autoimmune or infective diarrhoea leading to loss of mucosal integrity.
4. Dysmotility: altered gut motility related to drugs, recovery from ileus or pseudo-obstruction.

5. A recent stool culture is positive for *Clostridium difficile* (Cdiff). What are the risk factors for Cdiff infection? [3 for all]

Think in terms of three categories:

1. Factors that disturb endogenous intestinal flora/function:
   - Antibiotics (90% of hospital Cdiff is related to cephalosporin, quinolones, clindamycin use)
   - Gastric acid suppression (results are conflicting here and the mechanism by which a high gastric pH influences Cdiff infection rates is unclear because spores are resistant to gastric acidity anyway!)
   - Enteral feeding (especially post pyloric tubes), enemas, nasogastric tubes
   - Chemotherapy, radiotherapy, immunosuppression
   - Drugs causing gastro-intestinal stasis (should be avoided where possible in Cdiff infection)
2. Environmental exposure to Cdiff spores – the length of hospital stay increases risk of exposure to Cdiff.
3. Patient factors:
   - Age > 65 years
   - Inflammatory bowel disease (immunosuppressants/impaired mucosal function)
   - HIV/AIDS
   - Chronic kidney disease
   - Concomitant infection (sepsis, pneumonia, skin infection, UTI) – probably due to antibiotic use

6. What do you know about the pathophysiology of Cdiff diarrhoea? [2 for all]

Clostridium difficile is a Gram-positive, spore-forming bacteria.

It causes diarrhoea by secretion of exotoxins (A and B).

Both toxins cause neutrophilic infiltration of and damage to the colonic mucosa. The toxins disrupt the actin cytoskeleton of enterocytes leading to opening of tight junctions and leakage of fluid into the intestinal lumen. Hence it is an inflammatory form of diarrhoea.

An inflammatory slough may form over mucosal ulcerations creating the appearance of a pseudomembrane with is pathognomic for Cdiff infection.

7. What features are associated with severe Cdiff infection?   [3 for all]

There is no formal consensus regarding mild/moderate severe infection.

    However, as a guide:

- Mild/moderate infection: diarrhoea/abdominal cramping, no systemic symptoms
- Severe infection: abundant diarrhoea, abdominal pain, leukocytosis, fever or other systemic symptoms
- Fulminant infection: severe Cdiff plus peritonitis/perforation/ileus with toxic megacolon or the presence of shock (needing inotropes is a very poor sign)

Data 4

A 50-year-old lady is referred to you by the emergency department. She has been caught in a house fire and has been rescued by firemen. She is very drowsy and has suffered a suspected inhalational injury and also burns to her neck and thorax and legs.

1. The burns doctors have completed a chart to show the severity of her burns. What is the estimated total body surface area (BSA) involved?

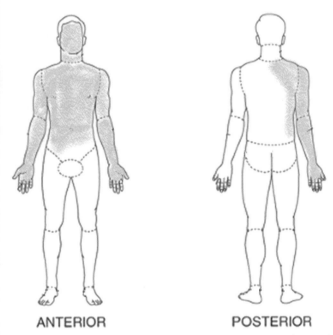

ANTERIOR   POSTERIOR

For the colour version, please refer to the plate section. In some formats this figure will only appear in black and white.

The rule of nines estimates this around 45% BSA, Lund–Browder estimates BSA at 37.5%. [2]

2. What systems are there available to help us estimate the percentage of burns (if not already named above)? [3 for all]

Systems available are the rule of nines, Lund–Browder diagrams or you can use the palm as 1% BSA for small burns. Diagrams are shown below for reference.

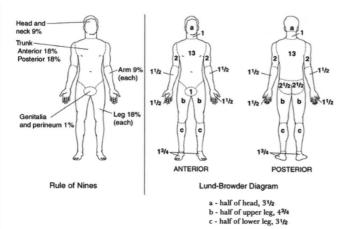

Head and neck 9%

Trunk
Anterior 18%
Posterior 18%

Arm 9% (each)

Genitalia and perineum 1%

Leg 18% (each)

Rule of Nines

13

1½   1½

1½   1½

ANTERIOR

13

1½   1½

2½ 2½

1½   1½

POSTERIOR

Lund-Browder Diagram

a - half of head, 3½
b - half of upper leg, 4¾
c - half of lower leg, 3½

3. What are the features you would be particularly looking for when assessing her airway? [2 for > 4]

The features to look out for are:

- Hoarse voice
- Stridor
- Soot in nose/mouth/airway
- Carbonaceous sputum
- Singeing of nasal hair
- Swelling of tongue, neck, airway

4. Can any investigations help?

Nasendoscopy may have a role, but it is usually fairly obvious that there has been a facial burn. Carboxyhaemoglobin levels on an arterial blood gas test can give an indication of the degree of smoke inhalation. [2]

5. What is carboxyhaemoglobin? Is it a problem? What levels should we be worried at? [3 for all]

Haemoglobin that has carbon monoxide (CO) bound to it instead of oxygen. Carbon monoxide's affinity for haemoglobin is 200 times stronger than for oxygen, effectively displacing oxygen from the haemoglobin molecule.

Carboxyhaemoglobin also contributes a slight artifactual increase in measured SpO_2 levels measured by oximetry. The effect is small, but becomes more marked as the true SpO_2 falls. Carboxyhaemoglobin levels of 45% will cause a 3–7% artifactual increase in measured SpO_2.

Normal carboxyhaemoglobin levels in the blood are from 1% to 3% of total haemoglobin. Overt toxic signs of carbon monoxide poisoning usually appear when carboxyhaemoglobin levels reach 15–20%. Levels over 40% are associated with agitation, confusion and shock. Blood carboxyhaemoglobin levels may underestimate the degree of CO intoxication because of oxygen administered to the patient before arrival to the hospital.

6. Does she need intubating? Why (not)? [1 for yes, 1 more for justification]

She has suffered a significant burn with likely smoke inhalation and facial involvement. Any concern for the airway, or potential for the airway to become swollen and difficult to manage should prompt intubation. Similarly, the need for aggressive fluid resuscitation and primary or secondary hypoxia as a result of the inhalation injury should prompt intubation, bronchoscopy and ventilation.

7. Are there any special considerations as you prepare to secure her airway?

She has a high chance of a difficult airway. Expertise and equipment to manage this situation in the emergency department must be available. An un-cut endotracheal tube is needed as the face is likely to swell once fluid resuscitation begins. Siting a nasogastric tube is also an early priority as this may quickly become very difficult. Massive tissue injury can be associated with hyperkalaemia associated with burns, although this tends to be more of a problem over the first few days post injury. This may affect your choice of neuromuscular blocker (not suxamethonium). [2]

8. How would you calculate her fluid requirements in the first 24 hours?

Parkland formula is a common example. 4 ml/kg lactated ringer's in the first 24 hours (half in the first 8 hours and the other half in the next 16 hours). [1]

This is a rough guide and must be supplemented by clinical and laboratory indicators.[1]

9. What factors would you consider when taking into account transfer to a burns centre? [2 for most]

The British Burns Association suggested minimum thresholds for referral into specialized burn care services. Examples include:

- All burns $\geq$ 2% total BSA in children or $\geq$ 3% in adults
- All full-thickness burns
- All circumferential burns
- Any burn not healed in 2 weeks
- Significant burns to special areas (hands, feet, face, genitalia)
- Significant mechanisms of injury such as blasts
- Significant co-morbidities that may affect wound healing
- Significant inhalation injuries

Data 5

A 40-year-old man was involved in a high-speed road traffic accident. He was the front-seat passenger when the car hit a tree. He was wearing a seatbelt. He is acutely short of breath. This is his chest X-ray.

1. **What abnormalities are seen on his admission chest X-ray?**

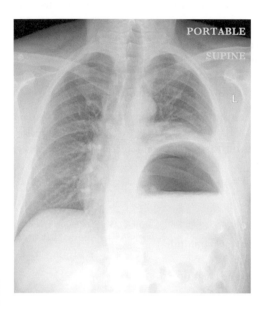

The chest X-ray shows an elevated left hemidiaphragm with a clear gastric 'bubble' and air–fluid interface in the stomach, which is inside the chest. The mediastinum appears displaced. [2]

2. **What are the possible causes for this abnormality?**

There are several possible causes for an elevated hemidiaphragm on a chest X-ray. It can either be 'pulled up' from above, 'pushed up' from below or be ruptured.

Given the history of severe trauma, the possibility of a possible phrenic nerve injury should be considered. [1]

Respiratory pathology including atelactasis and rib fractures can result in an elevated hemidiaphragm. [1]

Abdominal pathology including splenic injury, haematomas and subphrenic collections should also be considered. [1]

Finally, direct trauma to the diaphragm resulting in a diaphragmatic rupture is an important diagnosis to exclude and can be caused by either blunt or penetrating trauma. Most diaphragmatic injuries are on the left side. [2]

3. How would you confirm your suspicion of diaphragmatic injury?

A CT scan with contrast will be diagnostic. [1]

Classically, insertion of a nasogastric tube and its appearance in the left hemithorax is consistent with the diagnosis, although CT scanning is simpler and avoids worsening any potential gastric or oesophageal injuries. [1]

The diagnosis can also be confirmed with techniques such as laparascopy or thoracoscopy. [1]

Diaphragmatic rupture/tears are occasionally diagnosed coincidentally at laparotomy. [1]

4. How would you manage this complication?

The treatment is direct surgical repair through a laparotomy. [1]

Supportive treatment includes invasive ventilation and management of any associated injuries. [1]

5. Look at this CT scan taken in a trauma setting. What is the pathology? How would this be best managed?

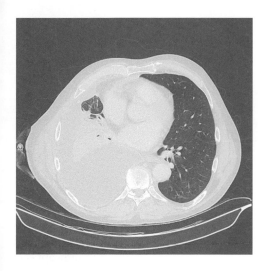

The CT scan of the chest shows a large fluid collection in the right hemithorax. This fluid is somewhat dependent and there is compressive atelectasis. The attenuation of the fluid makes this likely to be blood. [1]

This complication is best managed through the insertion of a large-bore chest drain and replacement of ongoing blood loss with blood and blood products (massive transfusion protocol). [2]

6. What are the indications for surgical intervention here?

A thoracotomy may be indicated if > 1.5 litres blood drained immediately, there is ongoing blood loss of 200–250 mL/hour over the next 4 hours or in the presence of haemodynamic instability. [2]

7. Describe how you will prepare for a chest drain insertion in this case.

[2 for all with structure]

Patient – Give an explanation and obtain consent. You need adequate intravenous access. Review the imaging and confirm correct side.

Equipment – You need adequate basic monitoring, and a formal chest drain insertion kit (scalpel, curved clamp, chest drains of various sizes, underwater seal). A Seldinger drain is not appropriate in the setting of a haemothorax.

Personnel – You need appropriate trained assistance.

Drugs – You need access to local anaesthesia, analgesia, oxygen if needed.

Identify landmarks – The 'safe triangle' describes an area bordered by the lateral border of the pectoralis major, the anterior border of the latismus dorsi and above the horizontal level of the nipple and with an apex below the axilla. The 5th intercostal space in the mid-axillary line is in this safe triangle.

Data 6

A 55-year-old man is brought into hospital post resuscitation for ventricular fibrillation (VF) arrest. There is return of spontaneous circulation (ROSC) after 20 minutes and his Glasgow Coma Scale (GCS) is 4/15. His ECG is provided.

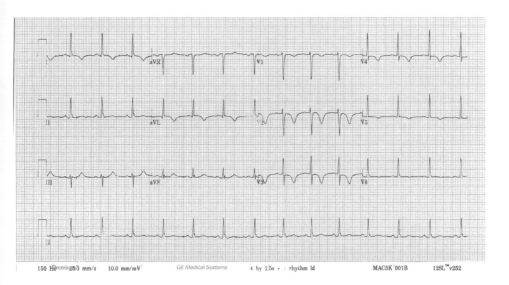

1. **Describe the ECG.**
The rate is approximately 80/min, sinus rhythm, normal axis, normal P morphology and PR interval, normal QRS complexes without Q waves but there is marked T-wave inversion anterolaterally (I, AVL, and across the V leads) implying anterolateral ischaemia.   [3]

2. **What broadly are the principles in your management?**
Important principles are assessment of the following:
- Airway – endotracheal intubation   [1 for all]
- Breathing – avoid hypo/hyperoxia; aim for normocapnia
- Circulation
- Disability – GCS and pupils
- Cardiovascular protection with early administration of antiplatelets   [1]
- Early revascularization (PCI) and haemodynamic support   [1]
- Neuro protection including targeted temperature management and maintenance of normoglycaemia   [1]

3. What target temperature would you aim for? Explain.

Consider target temperatures of 33 °C and 36 °C. You can argue a case for either. The TTM trial (*NEJM* 2013; 369: 2197–2206) showed that patients maintained at targets of 36 °C had similar outcomes to those maintained at 33 °C. Cooling is probably good, but perhaps not as important as ensuring that they don't get too hot. A recent advisory statement published by the International Liasion Committee on Resuscitation (ILCOR) recommends maintaining a constant target temperature between 32 °C and 36 °C.   [2]

4. How and when would you neuroprognosticate? What clinical features would help predict the likelihood of a poor outcome?

The consensus is that you wait at least 72 hours (if not longer) if targeted temperature management is used.   [1]

The following clinical signs all predict a poor neurological outcome for the cardiac arrest survivor, who has not undergone therapeutic hypothermia: absent pupillary or corneal reflexes and absent or extensor motor response and the presence of myoclonus, all at 72 hours. Cooling makes this time period effectively longer.   [3]

5. What other tests could you use – and what would you be looking for?

Electroencephalogram (EEG):

EEG features are associated with a poor outcome: generalized suppression, burst suppression and an isoelectric EEG. An EEG may demonstrate subclinical seizure activity.   [1]

Bispectral index (BIS):

A modified EEG is obtained by attaching a specially designed electrode to the head and gives a BIS value between 0 and 100, indicating the level of cerebral activity. A BIS value of 0 predicts a poor neurological outcome. BIS scores > 0 have limited prognostic value. Using suppression ratios alongside an actual BIS value may improve predictive capability.   [1]

Somatosensory-evoked potentials (SSEP):

A useful tool with a low false positive rate.

Evoked potentials are signals generated in the central nervous system after sensory stimulation. The main response normally seen is the 'N20' signal in the primary somatosensory cortex. This is a negative 'N' signal deflection 20 μs after electrical stimulation of the median nerve. Bilateral loss of this response indicates cortical cell death, provided that nerve function is intact at the brachial plexus.   [1]

Radiological:

CT scanning of the head is of limited value and is often useful to exclude an initial intracerebral event such as an intracerebral haemorrhage. Loss of grey–white matter differentiation has not been shown as a useful prognostic indicator of the long-term neurological outcome at an early stage.   [1]

Biochemical markers:

Certain biochemical entities are thought to indicate cerebral damage. These include neuronal specific enolase (NSE) and S-100b calcium binding protein. However, biomarkers are still largely a research tool. Raised levels, after cardiac arrest, are associated with the increased likelihood of a poor neurological outcome.   [1]

6. What scoring systems do you know of that can be used to assess neurological outcome post cardiac arrest? Describe one. [2]

Cerebral performance categories:

    CPC 1   Full recovery or mild disability

    CPC 2   Moderate disability but independant in activities of daily living

    CPC 3   Severe disability; dependent in activities of daily living

    CPC 4   Persistent vegetative state

    CPC 5   Dead

Glasgow Outcome Scale scoring system:

1. Death
2. Persistent vegetative state – severe damage with prolonged state of unresponsiveness and a lack of higher mental functions
3. Severe disability – severe injury with permanent need for help with daily living
4. Moderate disability – no need for assistance in everyday life, employment is possible but may require special equipment
5. Low disability – light damage with minor neurological and psychological deficits

Data 7

This is an image of a patient who is 5 days post emergency caesarean section. The patient complains of excruciating pain and has become febrile and hypotensive. You are asked to assess her.

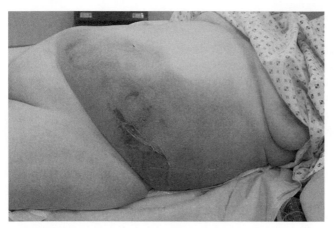

For the colour version, please refer to the plate section. In some formats this figure will only appear in black and white.

1. What does this picture demonstrate and what is the diagnosis?

It shows swollen, erythematous flank with evidence of blistering and skin necrosis. [1]

It shows necrotizing fasciitis – which is a life-threatening infection of the deeper dermal layers, subcutaneous tissue and fascial planes. [1]

2. Can you name some potential risk factors for necrotizing fasciitis?

[1 for each to a max. of 3]

Some risk factors are:
- History of trauma
- Immunosuppression, chronic illness
- Diabetes
- Cancer
- Drug abuse
- Alcoholism

3. Which organisms can cause this?

Most often group A streptococcal infection. [2]

Other organisms include *Staphylococcus aureus*, *Clostridium perfringens*, *Bacteroides fragilis*, *Aeromonas hydrophilia* and *Klebsiella pneumoniae* amongst others. [1 for > 3]

4. How would you manage this condition?

You would manage with the following:

- Aggressive resuscitation/sepsis bundles – likely to need vasopressors [1]
- Urgent surgical debridement [2]
- Early consultation with microbiology [1]
- High-dose intravenous antibiotics (clindamycin, benzyl penicillin + gentamicin as an example of an initial regime) [1]
- Intravenous immunoglobulin to combat toxin production [1]
- Referral to plastic surgical centre [1]
- Hyperbaric oxygen – controversial [1]

5. How can the surgical team manage the wound if it won't close?

Vacuum assisted closure (VAC) therapy can promote healing, help close wounds, or reduce the size of larger defects that would have been difficult to deal with. Reconstructive surgery should be considered only once the patient has been stabilized and the infection fully eradicated. [1]

6. Is there anything you could suggest to prevent further infection if the wounds extend around to the perineum and buttocks?

A defunctioning colostomy should be considered if wounds are regularly contaminated with faeces. [1]

7. Give examples of other infections that may be associated with group A streptococcus? [2 for >3]

Examples of infections are:

- Throat infections – tonsillitis, pharyngitis
- Skin infection – impetigo, cellulitis, erysipclas, scarlet fever
- Respiratory infections – pneumonia
- Invasive infections – necrotizing fasciitis, streptococcal toxic shock syndrome

Data 8

A 50-year-old woman presents to the emergency department with acute shortness of breath.

She has a past history of intravenous drug use but claims to have stopped using intravenous recreational drugs around 3 years ago. She has recently been diagnosed with 'angina' by her GP. She is drowsy and tachypnoeic with a GCS of 9 and a respiratory rate of 30 breaths per minute. An arterial blood gas test is consistent with type 1 respiratory failure.

Her chest X-ray on admission is shown below.

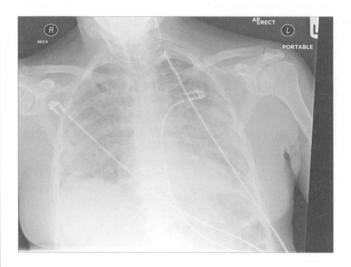

1. What is the differential diagnosis for the cause of her dyspnoea?   [2 for all]

Her dyspnoea may be caused by the following:
- Pneumonia – bacterial/atypical/viral/aspiration (low GCS)/opportunistic infection – e.g. pneumocystis carinii pneumonia (PCP) (technically this is *Pneumocystis jiroveci* (PCJ))
- Cardiogenic pulmonary oedema
- ARDS – primary or secondary
- Pulmonary embolism is a possibility

2. How would you define ARDS? Can you tell me what the Berlin definition of ARDS is (if not offered)?   [3 for all, 2 for most]

ARDS is an acute diffuse, inflammatory lung injury, leading to increased pulmonary vascular permeability, increased lung water and loss of aerated lung tissue. This leads to hypoxaemia and bilateral radiographic opacities, associated with increased venous admixture, increased physiological dead space and decreased lung compliance.

The Berlin definition (*JAMA* 2012; 307(23): 2526–2533) takes into account:

- *Timing* – Within 1 week of a known clinical insult or new or worsening respiratory symptoms
- *Chest imaging* – Bilateral opacities not fully explained by effusions, collapse or nodules
- *Origin of oedema* – Respiratory failure not fully explained by cardiac failure or fluid overload
- *Oxygenation* –

  Mild $PaO_2/FiO_2 \leq 200$ mmHg or ≤ 300 mmHg with PEEP or CPAP ≥ 5 cmH$_2$O

  Moderate $PaO_2/FiO_2 \leq 100$ mmHg or ≤ 200 mmHg with PEEP ≥ 5 cmH$_2$O

  Severe $PaO_2/FiO_2 \leq 100$ mmHg with PEEP ≥ 5 cmH$_2$O

3. She deteriorates and is admitted to critical care for intubation and ventilation. What settings would you put into the ventilator initially? Prompt if not offered ('What positive end expiratory pressure (PEEP)', etc.).

Suitable initial ventilator settings are the following:

- 6 ml/kg tidal volume (ideal body weight) [1]
- Limit plateau pressures (max. 30 cmH$_2$O), permissive hypercapnia [1]
- Pressure or volume control (no difference – although the ARDSnet study was based on volume-controlled ventilation). [1]
- Optimal PEEP (How would you set this?), look for a reasonable strategy (based on FiO$_2$ or inflection points of compliance curves) [1]

4. This is the pressure/time graph. What mode of ventilation is this?

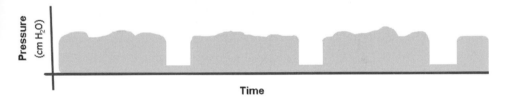

There is a markedly reversed I:E ratio (approximately 5 to 1) which would suggest airway pressure release ventilation (APRV) or a deliberate reverse I:E ratio strategy using conventional mandatory ventilation. [1]

5. What potential problems can this ventilatory strategy lead to?

Short expiratory times can lead to 'breath stacking' especially if there is airflow limitation or bronchospasm. Long periods of inspiration at high pressures can cause barotrauma or haemodynamic problems if underfilled. Hypercapnia can be a problem as effective minute volume is reduced, although this may be balanced over time with improved tidal volumes. [2]

6. You and your team consider that she is managed with appropriate ventilatory settings. Arterial blood gases on 100% FiO$_2$, pH 7.2, PaO$_2$ 7.5 kPa, PaCO$_2$ 7.8 kPa, HCO$_3^-$ 22. What would you do?

The management of refractory hypoxaemia involves the consideration of the following strategies: [1 each, up to max. 5]

- Conservative fluid management strategies (FAACT trial, *NEJM* 2006; 354: 2564–2575), including optimizing Hb and albumin levels
- Use of recruitment manoeuvres
- Muscle relaxants (*NEJM* 2010; 363(12): 1107–1116)
- Prone positioning
- High-frequency oscillation (OSCAR, *NEJM* 2013; 368(9): 806–813, showed no mortality benefit and the OSCILLATE trial showed worse outcomes with HFOV)
- Extra Corporeal Membrane Oxygenation (ECMO)–CESAR trial (Peek, *Lancet* 2009; 374(9698):1351–1363) demonstrated improved outcomes in patients transferred to an ECMO centre but not necessarily receiving ECMO
- Trials of inverse I:E ratios
- Trials of high PEEP

7. How does prone positioning work? [2 for all]

It works essentially by improving the ventilation/perfusion (V/Q) mismatch and reducing the shunt.

It shifts fluid from dorsal aspects of the lung, allowing alveoli to be recruited and improving ventilation to dependent areas.

There is less cardiac/abdominal compression and improved functional residual capacity (FRC).

Improved diaphragmatic function/homogenization of trans-pulmonary pressure gradients and mobilization of secretions all contribute to improved lung mechanics.

8. Which patients benefit most from prone positioning?

It is better for those with secondary ARDS (oedema and atelectasis) as compared to those with a pneumonia or lung consolidation. The PROSEVA trial (*NEJM* 2013; 368(23): 2159–2168) showed a survival benefit in severe ARDS. [1]

Data 9

A 72-year-old man has presented acutely to the emergency department with a 2-day history of difficulty in breathing which has markedly deteriorated over the last 4 hours. He lives alone and has been accompanied by a close friend.

His observations are as follows:

Respiratory rate – 30 breaths/minute
BP – 170/100 mmHg
Heart rate 110/min
SpO_2 94% on 40% FiO_2

He is barely able to talk and obviously struggling with his breathing and has evidence of severe inspiratory stridor and paradoxical breathing.

1. What are the possible causes for his presentation?
Differential diagnosis in an adult presenting with stridor would include:

[3 for all, 2 for most]

- Tumours – laryngeal/pharyngeal
- Extrinsic compression – goitre, mediastinal mass
- Vocal cord pathology – bilateral vocal cord paralysis, vocal cord dysfunction
- Infection – epiglottis (rare), tracheobronchitis
- Anaphylaxis – look for associated tongue/facial swelling
- Foreign body

2. How would you approach the management of this patient?
You need to assess airway patency. Ensure oxygen is connected and delivered. [2]
This man has severe stridor of as-yet indeterminate cause. Management at this stage would include administering an adrenaline nebulizer, intravenous hydrocortisone and seeking urgent ENT review and back-up. [2]
His airway is at risk and he has a potential difficult airway and needs experienced senior help, monitoring and difficult airway equipment at hand. If safe to do so, transfer to a more controlled environment such as the operating theatre should be actively considered, to allow securement of the airway and direct laryngoscopy. [2]
Tracheostomy under local anaesthesia may be a potential management option. [1]
Nasendoscopy in the emergency department is potentially hazardous and only performed by an experienced ENT surgeon along with adequate anaesthetic backup. [1]
Heliox (a mixture of 79% helium and 21% oxygen) is a low-density gas which reduces airway resistance and turbulence. Its role in this setting is at best temporizing and controversial especially given that this man is already hypoxic. [1]
Give intramuscular adrenaline and intravenous antihistamine if anaphylaxis is suspected. [1]

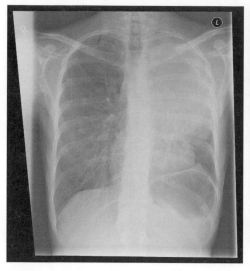
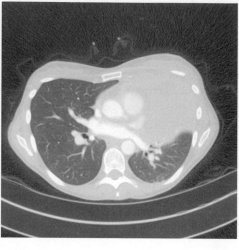

3. This man's condition dramatically stabilizes and this is a subsequent chest X-ray and CT image of his chest. What does this demonstrate? [2]

Imaging shows the presence of a mediastinal mass.

On the chest film there is a mass that occupies the left mid and upper zones. The left hemidiaphragm is pulled up and 'tented' implying volume loss.

The hilar vessels are seen through this mass, so it does not arise from the hilum and probably will arise from the anterior mediastinum.

The anterior location was confirmed on the corresponding CT image, with this slice at the level of the pulmonary trunk (highlighted by contrast).

Most commonly this will be a mass of thymic or lymphatic origin, although it is difficult to appreciate the exact origin of this mass from this CT slice alone.

4. What are the possible causes for this? [2 for all]

Possible causes are the following:

- Tumour – benign/malignant/metastasis, from lung, pleura, bone or distant spread
- Lymphoma
- Retrosternal goiter

5. Have you heard about NAP-4? Can you tell me in brief what this was about?

This is a national audit project conducted jointly by the Royal College of Anaesthetists and the Difficult Airway Society. This project looked into harmful events associated with airway management in theatre, intensive care unit and in the emergency department. [1]

Some themes emerging from this project included poor airway assessment, poor planning and a lack of airway management strategies. One in every four airway incidents arose either in the emergency department or intensive care unit. In the intensive care unit the lack of routine capnography significantly contributed to a large proportion of deaths and in the emergency department most complications occurred after rapid sequence induction. [2]

Data 10

A 50-year-old man had undergone a round of chemotherapy 18 months ago for lymph-oma. He was declared in remission some 12 months ago and had been well and returned to work as an office worker. He had been complaining of nausea for 3 weeks and went to his GP. Examination had been unremarkable but his blood urea and electrolytes (U&Es) were abnormal. He was sent to the medical admissions ward of your hospital and you are asked to see him by the on-call medical consultant because they are unsure as to how to treat him.

		Reference range
Sodium	109 mmol/L	136–145
Potassium	6.1 mmol/L	3.6–5.2
Urea	18.3 mmol/L	2.5–6.4
Creatinine	166 µmol/L	80–132
Chloride	81 mmol/L	95–105
Bicarbonate	12 mmol/L	22–28 mmol/L
WCC	10.9×10^9/L	4–11
Neutrophils	8.89×10^9/L	2–7.5
Haemoglobin	14.6 g/dL	11.5-16.5
Platelets	357×10^9/L	150–400
Total protein	58 g/l	64–82
Albumin	25 g/L	35–50
Globulin	33 g/L	23–35
Total bilirubin	30 g/L	3–17
AST	37 IU/L	15–37
Alkaline phosphatase	48 IU/L	50–136
Glucose	5.5 mmol/L	4.0–5.9
Calcium (corrected)	2.23 mmol/L	2.10–2.65 mmol/L
Phosphate	2.05 mmol/L	0.7–1.40 mmol/L
Magnesium	1.0 mmol/L	0.6–1.0 mmol/L

(cont.)

		Reference range
Amylase	107 IU/L	10–100 IU/L
LDH	516 IU/L	200–550 IU/L
INR	1.1	
APTT	30.3 seconds	28–38 seconds

1. What do you think of his laboratory results?

They show profound hyponatraemia with hyperkalaemia and hypochloraemia. [1]

They indicate metabolic acidosis with renal impairment. [1]

They show hypoalbuminaemia with slightly elevated bilirubin levels [1]

2. Why is sodium concentration so important? [2 for all]

It is the major extracellular cation in the body and the most important osmotically active
solute.

The ratio of sodium in intra- and extra-cellular fluid (the ICF–ECF ratio) is maintained by
the Na/K pump.

It influences the total body water volume and tonicity. Changes in sodium and tonicity
affect central nervous system cells.

3. How would you decide what the cause of his hyponatraemia is?

Since sodium and water can vary independently, low sodium can mean too little sodium,
too much water, or both. You need to do the following:

- Take a clinical history – e.g. of diarrhoea, diabetes, diuretics, fistulae [1]
- Perform a clinical examination – volume status [1]
- Carry out some laboratory investigations – serum/urine osmolarity and urinary sodium [1]

4. Can you classify hyponatraemia?

Hyponatraemia can be classified into hypertonic ECF, eutonic ECF and hypotonic ECF. [3]

- *Hypertonic ECF* : –
  - Water loss in excess of salt
    - Usually osmotic agent in plasma, e.g. mannitol or glucose
    - Not urea or alcohol as these go into both ECF and ICF
    - Low Na due to ICF water osmotically diluting ECF
- *Eutonic ECF*:
  - Usually spurious, e.g. hyper lipidaemia/proteinaemia
- *Hypotonic ECF (commonest)*:
  - You need an assessment of ECF volume – dry, euvolaemia or oedema
  - You need to assess whether the kidneys are handling salt and water appropriately
    (urinary sodium is usually enough)

Hypotonic hyponatraemia can be further classified based on an assessment of the volume
status. [3 if one example of each provided]

- *Hypotonic: oedema* – renal failure or fluid retention (congestive cardiac failure (CCF), liver failure):
  - . This is water excess
  - . Often patients are on diuretics (to treat)
  - . Renal retention of water is greater than that of sodium. Check urinary sodium:
    - – High urine Na > 20, kidneys failing to conserve salt – acute renal failure (ARF), chronic renal failure (CRF)
    - – Low urine Na < 10, usually with high urine osmolality >200 (concentrated); seen when water retention is in excess of salt retention, such as nephrotic syndrome, CCF or liver failure
- *Hypotonic: no oedema* – dilutional, e.g. syndrome of inappropriate antidiuretic hormone secretion (SIADH) or excess water in:
  - . Normal or slightly increased ECF volume (ECF is diluted)
  - . Kidneys unable to excrete water, i.e. can't excrete electrolyte-free water
  - . Urine osmolality inappropriately high >200 mmol/kg (often higher than plasma osmolality):
    - – Low urine Na, kidneys are excreting water but can't excrete enough – polydipsia, i.e. too much water in
    - – High Na, kidneys failing to excrete enough water. SIADH, hypothyroidism, Addison's disease
- *Hypotonic: dehydrated* – extra renal losses, cerebral salt-wasting syndrome (CSWS):
  - . Sodium loss and water loss but sodium >> water loss
  - . Hypovolaemia stimulates antidiuretic hormones (ADHs) and this over-rides the hypo-osmolar suppression of ADH secretion
  - . Renal water retention with concentrated urine:
    - – Low urinary Na (aldosterone stimulated by hypovolaemia):
      - Extra renal losses
      - - GI tract, skin, third spacing, peritonitis, ascities
    - – High urinary Na:
      - - Diuretic excess, salt-losing nephropathy, polyuric recovery, CSWS, mineralo-corticoid deficiency

5. Tell me about CSWS. [2 for all]

It is usually associated with subarachnoid haemorrhage (SAH).

Should the cause be unclear, remember that it can be related to atrial or brain natriuretic peptide (ANP or BNP) excess release.

It is characterized by renal sodium loss (with resultant water loss) together with hyponatraemia and hypovolaemia.

6. How would you differentiate it from SIADH? [2 for all]

It can be differentiated in the following ways:

- Excess urine output causing dehydration
- Very high urine Na >100 mmol/L (SIADH often > 20 mmol/L)
- Treatment of SIADH is fluid restriction
- Treatment of CSWS is fluid and Na resus:
  - . 0.9% Saline for correction is hypertonic
  - . In acute symptomatic states:

- – 3% Saline via central line but caution with too rapid correction
- – Frusemide if hypervolaemia occurs
- . Sometimes doesn't work
  - – Topping up Na drives further renal Na loss and associated further water loss

7. **What is the maximum rate of rise in sodium that you would aim for in a 24-hour period and what could happen if it rises too quickly?**

A maximum rate of rise of 10 mmols/day should be the aim. Too rapid a correction could result in the catastrophic consequence of central pontine myelinolysis. [2]

Related topics

SIADH:

- Described by Schwartz in 1957 with bronchogenic carcinoma
- Urinary sodium loss without corresponding water loss
- The ADH stops diuresis and causes water retention.
- Loss of control of ADH release. ADH concentration unchanged by drinking or osmotic stimuli
- Neurological (commonest)
  - . Meningitis/encephalitis
  - . Brain tumours
  - . SAH and traumatic brain injury (TBI)
  - . Neoplastic and non-neoplastic lung disease
  - . Drugs
- Treatment
  - . Water restriction
  - . Treat underlying cause
  - . Block action of ADH on collecting duct with demeclocycline or lithium

Diabetes insipidus (DI):

- Cranial (failure of ADH release) or nephrogenic (failure to respond to ADH)
- Commonly seen in brain death or injury
- Urinary excretion of water causing dehydration and hypernatraemia
- Cranial DI treated by DDAVP/desmopressin/vasopressin (replacing ADH) and water resuscitation

Data 11

You come onto the ITU for your shift and are asked what you would do about the bleeding chest drain that one of the trainees inserted earlier to treat a simple pneumothorax that occurred on a ventilator. There was a 1,000 mL haemorrhage which stopped within half an hour. The patient was taken for a CT thorax. The patient is sedated and ventilated still and the chest drain has stopped bleeding.

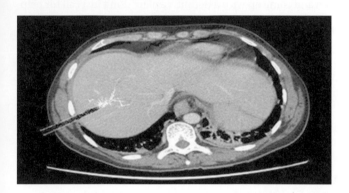

1. Comment on the CT.
The chest drain is clearly in the liver with some fresh bleeding. [1]
There is a residual pneumothorax. [1]

2. What would you do immediately? [2 for all]
You would discuss supportive measures and simple large-bore intravenous access, cross-match, resuscitation.
The patient still has an untreated pneumothorax and is on the ventilator.
The patient is likely to need a new chest drain.

3. How do you classify haemorrhagic shock and what would you expect to see clinically? [2 for all]
This is simplified from the Advanced Trauma Life Support (ATLS) training programme. It is important to note that sedated, ventilated patients will not show classic responses. There are four categories to consider:

Class I:	< 15% estimated blood loss (EBL) (750 mL)	Heart rate, blood pressure within normal range
Class II:	15–39% EBL (750–1,500 mL)	Tachycardia
Class III:	30–40% (1,500–2,000 mL)	Tachycardia, hypotension, hypoperfusion
Class IV:	> 40% (2,000 mL)	Marked hypotension and end organ failure

4. Would you give clotting factors?

You would only give clotting factors if indicated by laboratory abnormalities or following a massive transfusion. (NICE guidelines NG 24, Nov 2015) [1]

5. What are the options for management here? [3 for all, 2 for most]

Don't pull out the chest drain immediately.

Resuscitate and prepare for massive haemorrhage.

Seek expert assistance in considering laparotomy versus interventional radiology.

Potentially transfer the patient to theatre or even to another specialist centre.

Look for evidence of 'advanced' decisions – appreciate the risks and benefits of various strategies to manage the situation and come up with a definitive plan; don't just call for help.

6. What are the indications for a chest drain in general? [2 for most]

- Pneumothorax
  - in any ventilated patient
  - tension pneumothorax after initial needle relief
  - persistent or recurrent pneumothorax after simple aspiration
- Malignant pleural effusion
- Empyema and complicated parapneumonic pleural effusion
- Traumatic haemopneumothorax
- Post-operative – for example, thoracotomy, oesophagectomy, cardiac surgery

7. Where do you site a chest drain?

Insertion should be in the 'safe triangle' delineated by the anterior border of the latissimus dorsi, the lateral border of the pectoralis major muscle, a line superior to the horizontal level of the nipple and with an apex below the axilla. [2]

8. Discuss the pros and cons of the Seldinger vs. an open chest drain.

The Seldinger drain has less leakage, a smaller hole, it is adequate for less viscous fluids and air but is more likely to kink. [1]

An open drain has better pleural access, a bigger hole and drains complex collections or viscous fluids, such as pus or blood. [1]

9. What are the ultrasound features that would suggest a pneumothorax? [2 for most]

Ultrasound features include the following:

- Absence of lung sliding
- Absence of B lines
- Lung point
- Stratosphere sign

10. What precautions would you take with the intercostal drain during transfer?

[2 for most]

The drain should be properly secured.

The bottle should be kept upright at a lower level than insertion site and with an adequate underwater seal.

You should ensure it is free of kinks.

There needs to be suction tubing open to the air.

Appropriate monitoring is required.

Consider a Heimlich (flutter) valve.

Data 12

A 55-year-old man presents to the medics with recurrent pneumonias. They believe he has some sort of progressive muscular weakness, as yet undiagnosed. They ask you for your opinion regarding non-invasive respiratory support.

1. **What neuromuscular conditions could he have?**   [1 for categorization, 1 for at least 3 diagnoses]

Respiratory muscle weakness is common among patients who have neuromuscular disease. Respiratory failure can be acute (e.g. Guillain–Barré syndrome), chronic and relapsing (e.g. multiple sclerosis, myasthenia gravis), or progressive (e.g. amyotrophic lateral sclerosis, also commonly known as motor neurone disease in the UK). Conditions can also be classified by the location of the pathology either anatomically or functionally.

2. **In addition to history and examination, what tests can help us assess his respiratory status?**   [2 for all]

Appropriate tests are the following:
- Arterial blood gases
- Chest imaging – chest X-ray and possibly CT
- Pulmonary function tests (recognizing these are not always possible in acute illness)

3. **What information can we get from pulmonary function tests? How can they help us?**   [3 for all]

They can provide information on the following:
- Lung volumes and capacities
- Spirometry (FEV1, FVC values and peak flow)
- DLCO (transfer factor)

4. What do these flow-volume loops represent? (Blue line is normal reference)

[Score 1 for 2 correct, 2 for 3 or 4, 3 for all 5]

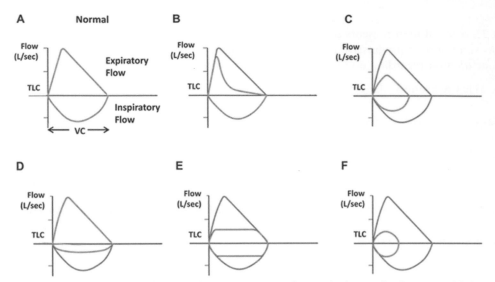

For the colour version, please refer to the plate section. In some formats this figure will only appear in black and white.

The loops represent the following:

A. Normal
B. Obstructive lung disease
C. Restrictive lung disease
D. Variable extrathoracic obstruction
E. Fixed upper-airway obstruction
F. Neuro-muscular weakness

5. How could DLCO help in this situation?

Diffusion capacity of the lung for carbon monoxide (DLCO), also known as the 'transfer factor' (TLCO), is a measurement of the ease of transfer for CO molecules from alveolar gas to the haemoglobin of the red blood cells in the pulmonary circulation. It often is helpful for evaluating the presence of possible parenchymal lung disease when spirometry and/or lung volume suggest a reduced vital capacity, RV, and/or total lung capacity. Interpretation can be complicated if there is reduced alveolar ventilation (VA) such as lung resection, restrictive lung defects, and so the DLCO:VA (KCO) ratio is often considered too. A reduced DLCO and a reduced DL-to-VA ratio suggest a true interstitial disease such as pulmonary fibrosis or pulmonary vascular disease. [2]

6. These are his pulmonary function tests. What do they represent?

		Reference range
FEV1	0.79 L (27% predicted)	3.17 L
FVC	0.87 L (22% predicted)	3.97 L
FEV1/FVC	91%	80%
FEV1 post bronchodilator	0.83 L	
TLCO	59% predicted	
KCO (10 seconds)	120% predicted	
VA	48% predicted	

These results show a low transfer factor, a high KCO but low VA suggesting poor chest expansion and respiratory muscle weakness. This is supported by the markedly reduced spirometry volumes. There is minimal reversibility post bronchodilator. [2]

7. What advice would you offer for his respiratory status?
An arterial blood gas test is needed to assess the respiratory function. The patient is likely to benefit from a trial of non-invasive ventilation. [1]
Physiotherapy input will be key and the use of devices such as cough-assist will be useful. [1]
You should treat any intercurrent infection. [1]
Assessment of bulbar function and swallowing status by speech and language therapists will help judge the risk of aspiration. [1]

8. Would you invasively ventilate him if he deteriorated?
[2 for answer with reasonable justification]
There is no clear answer at this stage as the diagnosis is not clear. It might be reasonable to ventilate whilst a diagnosis is made as there may be some reversibility. Patients with progressive neurological disease may not benefit from invasive ventilation, however, although this sensitive decision should be made after multidisciplinary input and discussion with the patient and their family.

Data 13

A 34-year-old, ex-intravenous drug user with a history of depression and back pain is admitted to your emergency department in an agitated state. His observations are recorded as follows:

Heart rate:	130 beats/min
Respiratory rate:	28 breaths/min
Blood pressure:	190/105 mmHg
Oxygen saturations:	98% (breathing room air)
Temperature:	40.1 °C

His regular medication includes the following:
- Diazepam, 2 mg QDS
- Methadone, 40 mg OD
- Citalopram, 10 mg OD
- Tramadol, 50–100 mg PRN
- Amitriptyline, 25 mg nocte

1. What are the potential causes of this patient's severe hyperthermia? [5 for all]
Potential causes are the following:
- Infectious causes
  . Potential sources include sepsis, CNS infection, endocarditis
- Environmental (heat stroke)
- Drug-related (bearing in mind that he may have taken anything!)
  . Serotonin syndrome
  . Withdrawal (e.g. alcohol, benzodiazepines)
  . Sympathomimetic toxicity (e.g. 'Ecstasy', cocaine)
  . Monoamine oxidase inihibitor (MAOI) toxicity
  . Neuroleptic malignant syndrome
  . Anticholinergic toxicity
  . Salicylate toxicity
- Endocrine disorders
  . Thyrotoxicosis
  . Phaeochromocytoma
- Central nervous system causes
  . Hypothalamic stroke

2. What are the cardiovascular consequences of untreated hyperthermia? [2 for all]
Hyperthermia affects all organ systems with increasing severity according to the duration of the hyperthermia and the extent of the temperature rise:

- Initial tachycardia and increase in stroke volume along with vasodilation and small decrease in mean arterial pressure
- Central venous pressure may fall as a consequence of fluid compartment shifting and dehydration
- As hyperthermia persists tachycardia may worsen. Metabolic acidosis leads to reduced myocardial contractility with decreased stroke volume and mean arterial pressure (MAP)
- Eventual hypotension and potential for myocardial infarction

3. What are the potential causes for his agitation/delirium? [2]

There are numerous causes which depend on the diagnosis:

- Direct drug effect (e.g. increased excitatory neurotransmitters)
- Metabolic derangement
- Drug or alcohol withdrawal
- Cerebral oedema (a consequence of hypertension and persistent hyperpyrexia)
- Cerebral haemorrhage/infarction (disseminated intravascular coagulation is a potential complication of hyperthermia)

4. What do you understand by the term serotonin syndrome? [3]

Serotonin syndrome describes the clinical features of dose-related, adverse effects of increased serotonin concentration in the central nervous system. There is a spectrum of severity ranging from mild through to life-threatening. Severe features only tend to occur in patients exposed to two or more serotonergic drugs. The diagnosis is clinical and the treatment is largely supportive. Mortality is low ($< 1\%$) with supportive care.

A classic triad of features may be observed:

a. Neuromuscular excitation (e.g. clonus, hyperreflexia, myoclonus, opsiclonus, rigidity)
b. Autonomic dysfunction (hyperthermia, tachycardia, mydriasis, flushing, sweating)
c. Central nervous system disturbance (anxiety, agitation, confusion, coma)

5. How is serotonin syndrome diagnosed?

The diagnosis is a clinical one and should be considered when features of serotonin syndrome are seen in the context of starting or increasing the dose of a known serotonergic drug or when a second serotonergic drug is added. [1]

6. Which drugs are known to cause serotonin syndrome? [up to 3 for classification and example for each category]

- *Drugs that prevent serotonin re-uptake or metabolism*
  - Selective serotonin re-uptake inhibitors (e.g. fluoxetine, citalopram)
  - Opioids (tramadol, pethidine)
  - Serotonin-noradrenaline re-uptake inhibitors (e.g. venlafaxine, duloxetine)
  - Mono-amine oxidase inhibitors (e.g. phenelzine, moclobemide but also linezolid and methylene blue)
  - Tricyclic antidepressants (e.g. amitriptyline, nortriptyline)
- *Drugs that stimulate serotonin release/serotonin agonists*
  - Opioids (tramadol)
  - 3,4-Methylenedioxymethamphetamine (MDMA or 'Ecstasy')
  - Amphetamines

- *Miscellaneous*
  - Lithium
  - Tryptophan
  - Buspyrone

7. What is the treatment for serotonin syndrome?   [2 for all]

Treatment is largely supportive, although critical care may be required in severe cases where severe hyperthermia, disseminated intravascular coagulation, ARDS and rhabdomyolysis may occur. In general:

- Stop the offending agent
- Sedation/control of agitation
- Active cooling (may ultimately require ventilation and paralysis)
- Control of heart rate and blood pressure
- Monitoring of coagulation and renal function

A number of specific treatments are available for severe serotonin syndrome although evidence as to their effectiveness is lacking (and may be difficult to obtain in a condition with a mortaliy of < 1% with standard treatment):

- Oral cyproheptadine (an oral $5HT_{2A}$ receptor antagonist)
- Intravenous chlorpromazine (risk of associated hypotension)

8. What techniques can be used for cooling in critical care?   [2 for all]

- *Passive techniques*:
  - Cool environment
  - Remove clothes/blankets
- *Active external cooling*:
  - Wet towels/ice packs/fans
  - Cooling blankets/pads
- *Active internal cooling*:
  - Cool intravenous fluids (4 °C)
  - Body cavity lavage (gastric, peritoneal, bladder, right pleural)
  - Extracorporeal (renal replacement circuit, cardiopulmonary bypass)

Comment

Many causes of fever are not causes of hyperthermia. The terms fever, hyperthermia and hyperpyrexia are used interchangeably although a stricter definition ought to apply:

- 'Fever' represents hypothalamic upregulation in response to infectious/non-infectious causes, as such it may be treated with antipyretics.
- 'Hyperthermia' represents failure of normal temperature regulation. It is not cytokine mediated and is unlikely to respond to antipyretics.
- 'Hyperpyrexia' is commonly used to refer to an extremely high temperature (> 41 °C).

Data 14

You are asked to review a 22-year-old, previously healthy, man who suffered a closed, isolated head injury. He has remained sedated and ventilated for 4 days to control his intracranial pressure and has remained relatively stable. The nursing staff describe him as being 'difficult to sedate'. His blood results are shown below.

		Reference range
Sodium	151 mmol/L	136–145 mmol/L
Potassium	5.6 mmol/L	3.6–5.2 mmol/L
Urea	7.1 mmol/L	2.5–6.4 mmol/L
Creatinine	163 µmol/L	80–132 µmol/L
Chloride	109 mmol/L	95–105 mmol/L
WCC	11.1×10^9/L	$4–11 \times 10^9$/L
Haemoglobin	15.0 g/dL	11.5–16.5 g/dL
Platelets	408×10^9/L	$150–400 \times 10^9$/L
Total protein	88 g/L	64–82 g/L
Albumin	44 g/L	35–50 g/L
Globulin	41 g/L	23–35 g/L
Total bilirubin	54 µmol/L	3–17 µmol/L
ALT	101 IU/L	30–65 IU/L
AST	222 IU/L	15–37 IU/L
Alkaline phosphatase	83 IU/L	50–136
Gamma GT	70 IU/L	15–85
Glucose	8.1 mmol/L	4.0–5.9
Creatinine kinase	4,432 IU/L	52–336 IU/L
FiO_2	0.45	
pH	7.31	7.35–7.45
pO_2	14.1 kPa	10.0–14 kPa
pCO_2	4.5 kPa	4.4–5.9 kPa
BE	–10.1 mEq/L	–2 – (+2) mEq/L
Lactate	3.1 mmol/L	0–2 mmol/L

1. Can you summarize the blood results?

The results indicate metabolic acidosis with a raised lactate and evidence of an acute kidney injury. There is what appears to be an acute liver injury and a markedly elevated creatinine kinase. Gas exchange is good. [2]

2. Tell me about lactic acidosis? [4 for all]

Lactic acidosis has been classified by Cohen and Woods. (The commonest . . .)

The commonest cause of a lactic acidosis is *type A*, hypoperfusion, and so haemodynamic data and optimization of perfusion is required first. *Type B* lactic acidosis occurs with normal perfusion, although occult tissue hypoperfusion is present in many cases. There are three B types:

- *Type B1*: Associated with underlying diseases (e.g. ketoacidosis, leukaemia, lymphoma, AIDS)
- *Type B2*: Associated with drugs and toxins (e.g. phenformin, cyanide, beta-agonists, methanol, nitroprusside infusion, ethanol intoxication in chronic alcoholics, anti-retroviral drugs)
- *Type B3*: Associated with inborn errors of metabolism (e.g. congenital forms of lactic acidosis with various enzyme defects (e.g. pyruvate dehydrogenase deficiency)

3. What can cause the raised creatinine kinase?

Muscular dystrophies, myositis, polymyositis, malignant hyperthermia, acute myocardial infarction, acute cerebrovascular disease or following neurosurgery intervention. Muscle breakdown is also seen in rhabdomyolysis, metabolic syndromes and hypothyroidism. [3]

4. He develops some bradycardias and this is his ECG. What do you make of it?

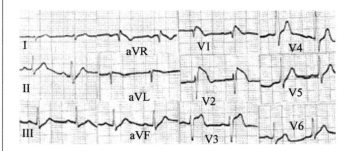

There is convex-curved ('coved') ST elevation in V1 to V3. [2]

5. Can you put all of this information together into a unifying diagnosis?

The ECG is classical for propofol infusion syndrome (PRIS). Right bundle branch block (RBBB) may be a feature. This ECG pattern usually precedes malignant ventricular arrhythmias in case reports of PRIS. This diagnosis is consistent with the metabolic acidosis, raised lactate and acute hepatic and renal derangement. [2]

6. Tell me about PRIS. [3 for all]

Most descriptions include acute refractory bradycardia leading to asystole, in the presence of one or more of the following: metabolic acidosis (base deficit > 10 mmol/L), rhabdomyolysis, hyperlipidaemia, and enlarged or fatty liver.

PRIS may be caused by either a direct mitochondrial respiratory chain inhibition or impaired mitochondrial fatty acid metabolism mediated by propofol. Predisposing factors seem to be young age, severe critical illness of central nervous system or respiratory origin, exogenous catecholamine or glucocorticoid administration, inadequate carbohydrate intake and subclinical mitochondrial disease.

7. Are there any other tests in addition to those you have seen already that would be useful?

Serum triglyceride levels can help with diagnosis. The patient needs to fast for 8–12 hours pre-test. High (200–499 mg/dL) or very high (500 mg/dL or above) levels are seen with lipaemic serum. [1]

8. What is the maximum dose of propofol recommended?

A typical maintenance range is 5–50 µg/kg per minute. There is an association between PRIS and propofol infusions at doses higher than 4 mg/kg per hour for greater than a 48-hour duration. [2]

9. How do you treat PRIS?

Treatment options are limited. Stopping propofol and using alternative sedation is needed. Haemodialysis or haemoperfusion with cardiorespiratory support have been the most successful treatment. An awareness of the syndrome and early recognition is key. [1]

Data 15

A 70-year-old man presents with rapidly developing ascending weakness following an episode of gastroenteritis. He is now referred to critical care with increasing dyspnoea and tachypnoea. Clinical examination confirms the presence of bilateral lower and upper limb weakness and diminished reflexes.

1. These are some test results. What test is this and what data is missing? What would you expect this to reveal? [2 for both]

	Sample	Normal range
Colour	Clear	Clear
White cells (per mm³)	2	< 5
Red cells (per mm³)	8	< 5
Plasma:glucose ratio	68%	66% (approx)

This is a cerebrospinal fluid (CSF) result and protein levels are missing, which are likely to be elevated.
Albumino-cytological dissociation is a feature of Guillain–Barré syndrome (GBS).

2. If the CSF protein is indeed high, what is the likely diagnosis?
He is likely to have GBS. [1]

3. Can you give some possible differential diagnosis for his weakness? [3 for a well-outlined structured approach with examples]
- Brainstem lesions – acute disseminated encephalomyelitis (ADEM)
- Spinal cord pathology – transverse myelitis
- Polyneuropathy –
  . Infective – polio, diphtheria, Lyme disease
  . Non-infective – acute intermittent porphyria
- Neuromuscular junction – myasthenia, botulism, diphtheria
- Muscle – rhabdomyolysis, myositis

4. What other specific investigations (apart from routine bloods) would you request to help make the diagnosis?
An MRI brain and cervical spine scan would rule out cord compression and brainstem lesions but you may need to intubate prior to this. [1]
You could carry out nerve conduction studies to differentiate demyelination from axonal damage. [1]
GBS can be associated with Campylobacter or viral infections. Test for antibodies for *Campylobacter jejuni*, a viral screen, mycoplasma serology, HIV testing, antiganglioside autoantibodies. [1]

5. What are the indications for intensive care admission? [3 for all]
- Respiratory failure, vital capacity < 15 mL/kg
- Bulbar weakness, inability to protect airway
- Autonomic instability – haemodynamic instability and cardiac arrhythmias

6. What intubation drugs would you use and why?
You would use an induction agent; titrate carefully as autonomic instability common. [1]
Make sure vasopressors and atropine are to hand (in case of severe bradycardia). [1]
Avoid suxamethonium, as this may induce hyperkalaemia. [1]

7. He is now intubated and cardiovascularly stable. What specific treatment measures would you consider? [2 for both]
Specific treatments are either intravenous immunoglobulin or plasmapheresis.
Both treatments are equally effective; the former is more expensive but is easier to administer and has fewer side effects than plasmapheresis.
There is no role for steroids.

8. What other supportive measures would you institute? [2 for all]
Management is largely supportive including:
- DVT prophylaxis
- Analgesic ladder/treatment of neuropathic pain
- Attention to nutrition/electrolytes and bowel management
- Physiotherapy and avoidance of pressure sores

Try and establish a means of communication. Use care bundles, such as a ventilator-associated pneumonia (VAP) reduction bundle.
   Tracheostomy is often indicated.

9. What is the prognosis?
The mortality for this condition is around 5%, with a significant proportion of survivors having significant permanent residual disability. The prognosis is worse in the elderly, in the presence of persistently poor neurology and where there is the need for prolonged mechanical ventilation. [1]

Data 16

Mr Smith is a 60-year-old male who is on the high-dependency unit 8 hours post elective laparotomy and small bowel resection with a large midline incision. He has a past history of stable angina and hypertension. He has an epidural *in situ* but is now complaining of peri-umbilical pain. His epidural infusion consists of Bupivacaine 0.1% and fentanyl 2 µg/mL running at 10 mL/hour.

This is his observations chart.

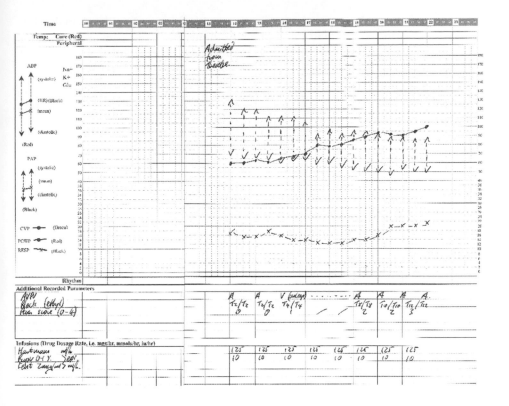

1. Tell me how you would assess this patient as regarding his current symptoms.

Take an adequate history: the site of pain, radiation, character and severity and any aggravating and relieving factors. [1]

Carry out an examination: blood pressure, heart rate, respiratory rate, SpO₂ (from the observation chart provided), capillary refill. [1]

Carry out an abdominal examination, including assessing the presence of any drain losses. [1]

Describe an assessment of the sensory level of analgesia using ethyl chloride spray and confirm that there is no significant motor block resulting from the epidural. [1]

Provide analgesia – consider an epidural top-up with a bolus dose of local anaesthetic, following correction of any hypotension, or provide alternative analgesia. [1]

2. What do you think of his blood pressure? What might have caused this?

The hypotension could be due to the sympathetic blockade caused by the epidural. [1]

Coexisting hypovolaemia is a strong possibility. [1]

Active ongoing blood loss needs to be excluded. [1]

An acute cardiac ischaemic episode also is a possibility here. [1]

3 What are the potential associated complications with the use of epidural analgesia?

- Risks related to insertion – post dural puncture headache, nerve damage at insertion, which may be transient or less likely permanent, epidural haematoma [1]
- Infective risks – epidural abcess [1]
- Risks related to pharmaceutical agents: [1 for both]
  . Local anaesthetic sympathetic blockade (hypotension, bradycardia) or motor blockade (weak legs)
  . Opiates (nausea, vomiting, pruritus)

4. What is the most important sign in a patient with suspected epidural haematoma?

Epidural haematomas can cause sensory and motor dysfunction, radicular pain and urinary retention. In the post-operative setting the most valuable sign is the presence of a motor block. If motor block is not reversible with cessation of the local anaesthetic solution (and pain/sensation returns implying that the analgesic effects have worn off) then suspicion of a haematoma should be high. [2]

5. How would you manage a patient with an epidural who has lower-limb weakness.

You should temporarily discontinue the epidural to assess sensory and motor function.[1]
You should substitute with other forms of analgesia in the interim. [1]
If motor or sensory signs persist proceed to obtaining an urgent MRI scan of the spine and seek urgent neurosurgical input. [2]

6. You have a patient with an epidural *in situ* who has inadvertently received two doses of clopidogrel. How would you manage this situation? [2 for all]

Discontinue further doses of clopidogrel.
Leave epidural catheter *in situ* at this stage.
You could consider performing a TEG/ROTEM/platelet function analysis to assess anti-platelet effects.
You need to fill in a critical incident form and inform patient.

Data 17

This is the chest X-ray of a young man who presents with fever, worsening shortness of breath and pleuritic chest pain.

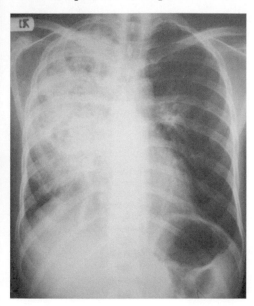

1. Describe the X-ray.
This is an adequate posterioranterior (PA) chest film of an un-intubated patient. There is a marked right-sided upper and middle zone consolidation with cavitation. [2]

2. Do you know of any scoring systems that can be used to assess the severity of this disease? – Elaborate. [1 for all]
The CURB-65 score could be used. The name is derived from the following:
- Confusion of new onset
- Urea greater than 7 mmol/L
- Respiratory rate of 30 breaths per minute or greater
- Blood pressure less than 90 mmHg systolic or diastolic blood pressure 60 mmHg or less
- Age **65** or older.

3. How is this score used for risk stratification? [1 for all]
The risk of death at 30 days increases as the score increases:
- 0 – 0.7%
- 1 – 3.2%
- 2 –13.0%

- 3 –17.0%
- 4 – 41.5%
- 5 – 57.0%

4. What first-line antibiotics would you use to treat severe community acquired pneumonia?

Local protocol usually involves a combination of a penicillin and a macrolide.   [1]

5. The patient is thought to be immunocompromised. What additional microbiological tests would you consider testing for in this situation?

Sputum/non-directed broncho-alveolar lavage (BAL) or formal BAL tests could be considered, including MC&S (microscopy, culture and sensitivity), AFB (acid-fast bacillus), aspergillus and other fungi, pneumocystis pneumonia (PCP)/HIV tests.   [2 for all]

If aspergillus is suspected check levels of galactomaman, beta D glucan in the blood and aspergillus precipitins and and carry out an IgG/IgE immunoglobin assessment.   [1]

6. What are the possible differential causes for lung cavitation?

- Bacterial pneumonia – caused by *Klebsiella pneumonia, Staphylococcus aureus* – especially PVL-producing strains (pneumococcal pneumonia usually does not cause cavitation)   [1]
- TB   [1]
- Aspiration   [1]
- Underlying immunodeficiency – (HIV) – cavities may be infective (TB/atypical mycobacterium/bacterial/invasive aspergillosis) or non-infective (NHL/Kaposi's)   [1]
- Non-infective causes of lung cavities include vasculitis, sarcoidosis, rheumatoid nodules, malignancy, pulmonary infarct   [1 for any]

7. Your microbiologist suspects a PVL-producing strain as a strong differential. What is PVL toxin? How does it present?

PVL is one of several extracellular cytotoxins produced by *S. aureus*. The toxin is leukocidal, destroying leukocytes by creating lytic pores in the cell membrane. It is most often associated with skin and soft-tissue infections and patients can occasionally present with pneumonia. [2]

8. What antibiotics would you use in this case and why?

[1 for correct antibiotics, 1 for explanation]

Early diagnosis is essential, as typical antimicrobial therapy for community-acquired pneumonia will not affect the PVL-toxin-producing strains. The microbiology laboratory must be involved early as specific investigations are required to guide therapy.

A significant proportion of PVL-positive clinical isolates of *S. aureus* causing pneumonia are methicillin-resistant so empirical therapy must cover MRSA.

The Department of Health has produced guidance on initial treatment and recommends linezolid 600 mg 12-hourly and high-dose clindamycin 1.2–1.8 g 6-hourly in combination, which may be synergistic. There have been many different regimes described, with the addition of rifampicin 600 mg twice daily to linezolid and clindamycin, probably being the most beneficial.

As the toxin continues to be active even if the bacteria can be successfully killed, adjunctive therapy can be used to attempt to inactivate the toxin.

Intravenous immunoglobulin should be considered as it may be partly effective in neutralizing super-antigens and toxins.   [1]

9. Is there a role for CPAP/NIV in the treatment of a severe community acquired pneumonia?

In short, there is very little evidence that continuous positive airway pressure prevents intubation and ventilation and may worsen the outcome if intubation is delayed when advanced respiratory support is inevitable. It may be reasonable to trial non-invasive ventilation (NIV) but only in a setting where intermittent positive pressure ventilation (IPPV) can be rapidly commenced, as a holding measure in the high-dependency-unit setting pre-intubation, or as the ceiling of treatment. [2]

Data 18

A 52-year-old woman is admitted to hospital with a 2-day history of being generally unwell, with fever and rigors. She has a background history of severe multiple sclerosis which has left her severely debilitated and fully dependent on her husband and carers for help with activities of daily living (ADLs) and with a long-term urinary catheter. Her husband describes her quality of life as poor. She remains hypotensive after having had 2 litres of crystalloid and is confused. She has demonstrable left-loin tenderness on clinical examination.

Her observations are as follows: blood pressure 70/40 mmHg, heart rate 96/min, capillary refill 4 seconds, oxygen saturation 92% on 10 litres, respiratory rate 22 breaths per minute. She has a Glasgow Coma Score of 14/15.

		Reference range
Sodium	132 mmol/L	136–145 mmol/L
Potassium	5.5 mmol/L	3.6–5.2 mmol/L
Urea	25.8 mmol/L	2.5–6.4 mmol/L
Creatinine	357 µmol/L	80–132 µmol/L
WCC	3.0×10^9/L	$4–11 \times 10^9$/L
Haemoglobin	11.3 g/dL	11.5–16.5 g/dL
Platelets	90×10^9/L	$150–400 \times 10^9$/L
Albumin	32 g/L	35–50 g/L
Total bilirubin	31 µmol/L	3–17 µmol/L
AST	76 IU/L	15–37 IU/L
Alkaline Phosphatase	88 IU/L	50–136 IU/L
Glucose	6 mmol/L	4.0–5.9 mmol/L
INR	1.4	
FiO_2	0.7 (approx)	
pH	7.3	7.35–7.45
pO_2	9.1 kPa	10.0–14 kPa
pCO_2	3.3 kPa	4.4–5.9 kPa
Bicarbonate	15.1 mmol/L	22–28 mmol/L
Lactate	4.6 mmol/L	0–2 mmol/L

1. What do you think is going on? [2 for both]

The clinical features are consistent with sepsis, possibly secondary to a urinary-tract infection (UTI).

The respiratory failure may be secondary to acute lung injury or pneumonia.

2. Are there any other bedside investigations or imaging that could be immediately helpful?

- Urine dipstix [1]
- Arterial blood gas test [1]
- Chest X-ray [1]
- Ultrasound scan (USS) of kidneys [1]

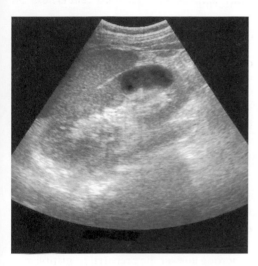

3. What does the ultrasound scan show?

There is a well-defined hypoechoic area within the cortex, which is typical of a renal abscess. Internal echoes within the parenchyma associated with a diffusely hypoechoic kidney, possibly resulting from acute pyelonephritis, may be seen. A perinephric (hypoechoic) collection may also be seen. [1]

4. What is sepsis?

A: A patient with suspected infection, a quick sequential organ failure assessment (SOFA) score $\geq$ 2 and evidence of organ dysfunction (SOFA score $\geq$ 2). The quick SOFA takes into account respiratory status, mental status and systolic blood pressure. *JAMA* 2016; 315(8): 801–810. [1]

5. What variables are indicated in the SOFA score?

A: These variables are the PaO_2/FiO_2 ratio, GCS, mean arterial pressure (MAP), vasopressor use, serum creatinine or urine output, bilirubin and platelet count. [2]

6. How do you define septic shock? [2 for all]

A: This is defined as shock where, despite adequate fluid resuscitation, vasopressors are required to keep MAP pressure $\geq$ 65 mmHg and serum lactate is > 2 mmol/L. [2]

7. What are the goals of treatment in the first 3 hours? [2 for all]

Use the sepsis 3-hour resuscitation bundle:

- Fluid challenge – 30 mL/kg crystalloid
- Blood cultures
- Check lactate levels
- Early antibiotics – within 1 hour of diagnosis

Also give oxygen to maintain saturation > 94%, monitor urine output and don't forget source control.

8. What are the goals of treatment in critical care? [2 for all]

- Fluid resuscitation titrated with dynamic monitoring
- Vasopressors to maintain MAP $\geq$ 65 mmHg
- Optimize delivery of oxygen using inotropes if required
- Aim to normalize lactate levels.

9. Are you aware of any trials that have informed the new Surviving Sepsis guidelines?

Three recent trials – PROCESS, ARISE and PROMISE – all failed to show a mortality benefit of early goal directed therapy (EGDT) as compared to standard care. There have undoubtedly been significant improvements in sepsis-related mortality over the last few years in large part due to better recognition and more effective earlier management. The utility of using an algorithmic EGDT approach, however, has now been called into question.

[2]

10. Eight hours later her condition continues to deteriorate and she remains on high-dose vasopressors and develops worsening renal failure now requiring haemofiltration. Would you consider this intervention as appropriate given the comments her husband made earlier? [2 for both]

This is an ethical question, which has no right or wrong answer. Be prepared to justify your answer on the limited information provided.

Progressive multiorgan failure in this setting is, however, associated with a significant increase in mortality. Any interventions would have to be carefully balanced and take into account benefits versus risks and burdens/level of distress caused; consider especially the patient's prior views, if known.

Data 19

This is the chest X-ray of a 35-year-old man admitted to the neurological intensive care unit with a severe head injury. He has been intubated for 4 days and now has increasing oxygen requirements.

1. **Can you comment on the chest X-ray. His chest X-ray on admission was reported as being normal.**

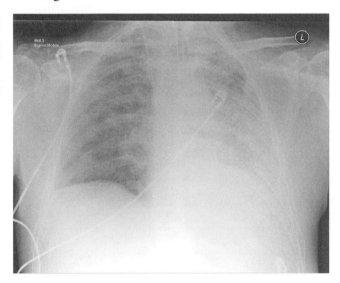

This shows a supine, mobile, adequate chest film of a patient who has got ECG monitoring and a right internal jugular central venous catheter (RIJ CVC) in an appropriate position. The most obvious abnormality is a dense opacification of the left lower zone, likely left lower lobar consolidation, presumably pneumonia. [2]

2. **Can you tell me a likely cause for this appearance.**

This man is likely to have developed a ventilator-associated pneumonia (VAP). [1]

3. **How do we diagnose VAP?**

The patient needs to have been ventilated for 48 hours. [1]

Clinical diagnosis is based on a combination of clinical signs, laboratory tests and chest X-ray interpretation. [1]

There are various scoring systems in use including the Clinical Pulmonary Infection Score (CIPS) and the CDC (US Center for Disease Control) and HELICS (Hospitals in Europe Link for Infection Control through Surveillance) definitions. [1]

4. **Can you tell me what elements are taken into account when calculating the CPIS score. What are the limitation of using this?**

There are five components of the CPIS score. They are: temperature, white cell count, oxygenation (PaO_2/FiO_2 ratio), character of tracheal secretions and chest X-ray features. [2]

Both clinical diagnosis and VAP scoring systems have limited diagnostic utility due to a lack of sensitivity and specificity.

5. What do you understand by the term ventilator-associated event?

The term ventilator-associated event (VAE) was coined to overcome the poor specificity and sensitivity of existing methods used in diagnosing VAP. Significant events or conditions (infective or non-infective) result in a deterioration in oxygenation ($> 20\%$ increase in the daily minimum FiO_2 or an increase in positive end expiratory pressure (PEEP) of at least 3 cmH$_2$O to maintain oxygenation from a previously stable baseline of at least 2 days).   [2]

6. What are the common organisms that cause a VAP?

- Gram-negative organisms – *Pseudomonas*, *Acinetobacter*, *Enterobacter*, *Klebsiella* and *Haemophilus* groups   [1]
- Gram-positive organisms – *Staphylococcus aureus*, *Streptococcus*   [1]
- Fungi – rare

7. What preventative measures can we use on an intensive care unit to reduce the incidence of VAP?

We can use bundles of care including good mouth care and ventilation bundles.   [1]

Components of a ventilation bundle include daily sedation holds, 30 degrees head up, chlorhexidine mouth care, sub-glottic suction and the use of humidification.   [1]

Selective decontamination of the digestive tract (SDD) may have a role to play in preventing VAP but is not in widespread clinical use.   [1]

8. What factors would you wish to take into consideration when deciding on appropriate antimicrobial therapy in treating VAP?

The choice of antibiotics would depend on local policy and knowledge of local pathogens. The local prevalence of multi-drug-resistant organisms, extended-spectrum beta-lactamase (ESBL) enzymes and methicillin-resistant *Staphylococcus aureus* (MRSA) should be taken into account.   [1]

Prior antibiotic therapy, a history of allergy and the duration of mechanical ventilation should also be considered. In general, early VAPs are caused by antibiotic-sensitive organisms whereas late-onset VAP is associated with drug-resistant organisms.   [1]

The results of any microbiological tests including broncho-alveolar lavage (BAL) results should be kept under review and early de-escalation based on the microbiological results considered.   [1]

9. Microbiological samples confirm MRSA in sputum. Which antibiotics would you consider using in this setting?

The glycopeptide antibiotic 'vancomycin' and the oxazolidinone 'linezolid' are the two most commonly used antibiotics currently available to treat an MRSA VAP. Current evidence on which is superior is conflicting. Undoubtedly, linezolid has better lung penetrance and some studies have reported better 'cure rates' associated with its use when compared to vancomycin. This, however, remains questionable and no study as such has demonstrated any mortality benefit when compared to vancomycin.   [2]

It is important, however, when using vancomycin, to take into account renal function and monitor trough levels, aiming for levels between 15 and 20 µg/mL. Some *S. aureus* isolates may show reduced sensitivity or indeed resistance to vancomycin.

Data 20

A 30-year-old man with a history of chronic alcoholism is admitted to critical care with a severe community acquired pneumonia. He is currently ventilated and on 0.20 µg/kg per minute noradrenaline and is due to commence enteral feeding. He has a body weight of 35 kg and a body mass index (BMI) of 15.

1. **What methods could you use to help calculate daily energy requirements for a patient in critical care?**

In general, the daily total energy requirements are calculated at 25–30 kcal/kg ideal body weight (IBW) per day as a rough estimate, or even lower, 20–25 kcal/kg, during the acute phase of illness. [2]

Daily protein requirements are estimated at 1.2–1.5 g/kg per day, which are included as part of the total energy requirements.

Calculating calorie requirements using predictive equations based on factors such as age, gender, height and weight are also recognized methods. Examples include the Harris–Benedict and Schofield equations. [1]

Indirect calorimetry may be a valuable tool to estimate energy requirements but is not widely available. [1]

2. **What nutritional problems may you expect to encounter specifically in this case?**

This patient appears to be severely malnourished. He is at risk of both over- and underfeeding and also is at risk of refeeding syndrome. [2]

3. **You calculate his daily protein requirements to be 50 g/day, how much energy does this provide? How much energy is provided by an equivalent amount of carbohydrate and fat?**

One gram of protein = 4 kcal, hence 50 g = 200 kcal. [1]

Similarly, a gram of carbohydrate = 4 kcal, hence 50 gms = 200 kcal. [1]

A gram of fat provides 9 kcal, hence 50 g fat = 450 kcal. [1]

4. **What do you understand by the term respiratory quotient (RQ)? What is the RQ for carbohydrates, fat and protein?**

$RQ = CO_2$ produced$/O_2$ consumed. [1]

For carbohydrates, RQ = 1.0.

For fats, RQ = 0.7 and for protein RQ = 0.8. [1]

5. **What is refeeding syndrome and what features would you look out for?**

Refeeding syndrome is a term used to describe the constellation of features that result from too rapid institution of feed in patients who have been food-deprived. [2]

Starvation is characterized by a shift from carbohydrate metabolism to fat and protein breakdown. Reinstituting feeds in such individuals causes a surge in insulin release and a rapid shift of electrolytes such as K^+, PO_4^- and Mg^+ into intracellular compartments. There may also be alterations in glucose homeostasis, thiamine deficiency and salt and water retention.

Life-threatening clinical features include severe muscle weakness, respiratory failure, cardiac dysrythmias, hypotension, heart failure, coma and death. [2]

6. How can you prevent refeeding syndrome?

Allow careful introduction of feed at lower rates in at-risk groups, e.g. at 10 kcal/kg per day to begin with, gradually increasing this as appropriate over several days. [1]

Ensure daily monitoring of fluid balance and electrolyte status, especially monitoring for hypokalaemia, hypophosphataemia and hypomagnesaemia and administer early replacement. [1]

Use multivitamin preparations (specifically thiamine). [1]

Note that the early input from a dietician is essential.

7. Apart from low body mass index (BMI), what are other risk factors for refeeding syndrome? [2 for all]

Other risk factors include:

- A history of unintentional weight loss greater than 10% in the last 3–6 months
- Poor nutritional intake for > 5 days
- A history of drug or alcohol abuse

Further additional information, refer to the NICE guidelines [CG32] published in February 2006.

Data 21

A 66-year-old gentleman was admitted with chest pain and diagnosed with an acute myocardial infarction (MI). He is acutely short of breath and you are asked to see him.

1. This is his chest X-ray. What does it demonstrate?

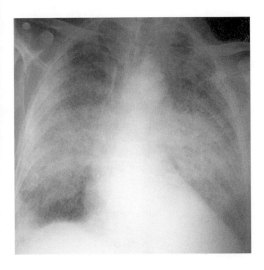

The chest X-ray shows extensive bilateral perihilar (bat's wing) oedema. This is classical case of acute pulmonary oedema. [1]

The short horizontal lines reaching the lung edge are 'Kerley B' lines and represent interstitial oedema. [1]

2. **This is a transthoracic echocardiogram (TTE) done soon after admission. Which view is this? The arrows point to regions which display wall motion abnormalities. Which wall is affected?** [2 for both]

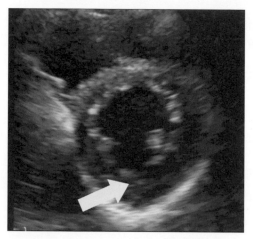

For the colour version, please refer to the plate section. In some formats this figure will only appear in black and white.

The TTE shows the parasternal mid short axis cut through both ventricles at the mid papillary muscle level.

The arrow is pointing to the inferior wall.

3. **This is another view taken in the same patient in systole. What view is this? What pathology is evident?**

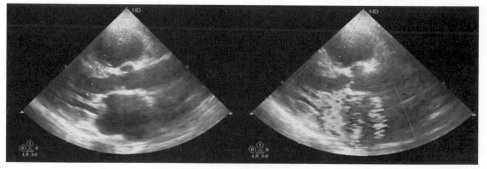

For the colour version, please refer to the plate section. In some formats this figure will only appear in black and white.

This is a parasternal long axis view, one with colour flow mapping. [1]

There is severe mitral regurgitation seen on the colour flow in the left atrium. There is a flail mitral valve seen prolapsing into the left atrium probably caused by a papillary muscle rupture. [2]

4. Which vascular territory is likely involved?

The TTE demonstrates inferior wall motion abnormalities. The inferior wall is usually supplied by the right coronary artery (RCA). [1]

There are two papillary muscles, the posteromedial and anterolateral. The former has only a single blood supply via the posterior descending artery (a branch of the RCA in 85% of patients and of the circumflex in 15%) and is the muscle most likely to be involved. [1]

5. What specific medical management strategies would you consider immediately instituting?

Medical management of this patient's pulmonary oedema would include the use of oxygen, intravenous frusemide, nitrates (if blood pressure allows) and CPAP. [2]

In addition, standard treatment of his acute MI with dual antiplatelet agents and heparin should be instituted. [2]

Consideration revascularization with urgent coronary angiography +/– stent insertion.
[1]

6. The pulmonary oedema remains refractory to the above management. What other options are available?

An intra-aortic balloon pump may have a role by causing a reduction of afterload and increasing cardiac output and by also improving diastolic perfusion of the heart. [2]

Expedient surgical management with either a mitral valve repair or replacement +/– coronary artery bypass grafting (CABG) may be an option for patients failing medical management and needs early discussion with a cardiothoracic surgeon. [2]

7. Apart from nitrates, can you name some other classes of drugs with vasodilating properties, which may have a role in the management of acute heart failure. [2 for most]

Other classes of drugs include the following:
- Phospho diesterase inhibitors – e.g. enoximone and milrinone
- Angiotensin-converting enzyme (ACE) inhibitors – e.g. ramipril, enalapril, perindopril
- Inotropes – e.g. dobutamine
- Calcium sensiters – e.g. levosimendan
- Miscellaneous – e.g. hydralizine, sodium nitroprusside

Data 22

You have been asked to assess a lady who is 35-weeks pregnant. She presented to the obstetricians with a one week history of feeling increasingly unwell, with a severe headache, fatigue, nausea and easy bruising. Blood tests are outlined below.

		Reference range
Sodium	134 mmol/L	136–145 mmol/L
Potassium	6.1 mmol/L	3.6–5.2 mmol/L
Urea	38.7 mmol/L	2.5–6.4 mmol/L
Creatinine	756 µmol/L	80–132 µmol/L
WCC	14.5×10^9/L	$4–11 \times 10^9$/L
Haemoglobin	7.5 g/dL	11.5–16.5 g/dL
Platelets	45×10^9/L	$150–400 \times 10^9$/L

1. **What are the possible differential diagnoses that could explain all the above abnormalities?** [2 for TTP, 2 for others as below]

The combination of anaemia, thrombocytopenia, neurological symptoms and acute kidney injury in pregnancy suggests a possible microangiopathic haemolytic process.

The differentials for this include thrombotic thrombocytopenic purpura (TTP), haemolysis elevated liver enzymes and low platelet count (HELLP) syndrome, eclampsia and haemolytic uraemic syndrome (HUS).

Other possible causes include autoimmune disease, infections (cytomegalovirus (CMV) infection, herpes simplex virus (HSV), HIV, hepatitis B), sepsis, vasculitis and drug induced causes.

2. **How would you confirm active ongoing haemolysis?** [3 for all, 2 for most]

A peripheral blood smear will show evidence of haemolysis:
- Fragments of the red blood cells (RBCs) (schistocytes) can be present
- There may be smaller and rounder RBCs (spherocytes)

There is a high reticulocyte count (immature red cells are released early as replacement).

There are low haptoglobin levels (this serum protein binds to free haemoglobin liberated from lysed cells).

The LDH levels are high.

There are elevated bilirubin levels (from RBC breakdown) and bilirubin breakdown products can be detected in the urine (e.g. urobilinogen).

3. **What confirmatory tests would suggest a diagnosis of TTP?** [1 for all]

Confirmatory tests include testing for levels of the protease enzyme ADAMTS13, which is often markedly reduced in sporadic cases of TTP.

Coombs tests (*direct* testing for antibodies or compliment proteins attached to the RBC membrane or *indirect* test for serum antibodies) are negative in TTP.

TTP and HUS differ mainly in the relative degree of renal failure. Typically, disorders in adults are described as TTP and are less likely to involve renal failure, but more likely to present with neurological abnormalities.

4. What is the pathophysiology involved in TTP?
ADAMTS13 enzyme is responsible for cleaving Von Willebrand (VW) factor. It can be congenitally absent (2–3%) or it can be reduced by an acquired autoimmune process. This is usually triggered by acute haemorrhagic colitis (Shiga toxin-producing bacteria such as *Escherichia coli* O157:H7, some strains of *Shigella dysenteriae*) although some chemotherapies and immunosuppressants can also trigger the disease. Large multimers of VW factor cause spontaneous platelet aggregation and subsequent haemolysis in the small vessels. [2]

5. What other investigations would you like to order? [3 for most]
- Clotting profile and liver function tests
- Autoimmune screen (antinuclear antibodies, rheumatoid factor, complement C3 and C4, cryoglobulins, serum immunoglobulins, antineutrophil cytoplasmic antibodies (ANCAs) and C-reactive protein (CRP))
- Appropriate culture looking for sepsis
- Renal and foetal ultrasound scan (intra-uterine growth retardation and death are associated)
- Cardiotocography (CTG) assessment of foetus in close liaison with obstetricians

6. What is the definitive therapy for this disorder?
The following are recommended:
- Early delivery of foetus if possible [1]
- Infusions of fresh frozen plasma (FFP) are a temporizing measure [1]
- Plasma exchange allows removal of auto antibodies and replenishment of enzyme levels [1]
- Intravenous methyl prednisolone in certain cases [1]

All the above are initiated after close discussions with haematologists and obstetricians with a special interest in this area.

7. What are the risks with haemofiltration in this case?
There are risks of vascular access, anticoagulation and intra-uterine bleed. [1]

8. Describe the process of plasma exchange? What are the potential complications? [2]
Blood is drawn and cellular components are separated from the plasma, either by centrifuge or filtration. The patient's plasma is then substituted with either fresh donor plasma or human albumin solution. Potential complications include bleeding, infection, allergic reactions, fluid overload and hypocalcaemia secondary to infused citrate.

9. Name some other indications for the use of plasma exchange in critical care [1]
- Neurological conditions include GB syndrome, Myasthenia Gravis, and chronic inflammatory demyelinating polyneuropathy.
- Renal conditions include Goodpasture's syndrome or ANCA associated vasculitis.

Data 23

A 45-year-old man presents with sudden collapse, seizures and a low Glasgow Coma Scale (GCS) of 3/15. This is his CT scan.

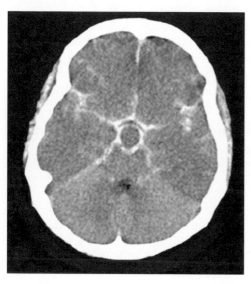

1. Describe the CT findings

The scan shows a swollen brain with loss of grey white differentiation. [2]

There is widespread sulcal and cisternal white hyperdensity (fresh blood).

2. What is the diagnosis?

The patient has suffered a subarachnoid haemorrhage. [1]

3. What is your immediate priority in management?

Check airway, breathing and circulation with particular emphasis on securing a definitive airway with early rapid sequence intubation, avoiding hypotension. [1]

4. What drugs would you use to aid intubation? [2 for all]

Thiopentone as an induction agent is the classical choice as reduces intracranial pressure.

Propofol is a reasonable alternative – most trainees will be more experienced or more comfortable with propofol and this may lead to more predictable haemodynamic changes.

Suxamethonium or rocuronium may be used for muscle relaxation.

A short-acting opiod or remifentanil infusion can be used to blunt the sympathetic response to intubation.

Metaraminol (or similar vasopressor) may be titrated to maintain the mean arterial pressure (MAP).

5. What other treatment measures would you take? [3 for all/2 for most]

Avoid secondary brain injury.

Balance need for maintaining cerebral perfusion vs. risk of rebleed. Current European guidelines suggest aiming for systolic BP <180 mmHg until coiling or clipping.

Ventilate to normocapnia.

Avoid hypoxia.

Ensure normoglycaemia.

Treat seizures.

Arrange urgent transfer to a specialist neurosurgical centre if appropriate.

6. What are the possible causes for this presentation?

Approximately 85% of cases of SAH are related to spontaneous rupture of an intracranial aneurysm. Non-aneurysmal bleeds account for 10% of cases. A further 5% include miscellaneous causes such as trauma or arteriovenous (AV) malformations. [2]

7. How would you grade its severity? [2 for all]

Severity is graded according to the World Federation of Neurosurgeons (WFNS) classification:

- Grade 1: GCS 15 and no motor deficit
- Grade 2: GCS 14–13 and no motor deficit
- Grade 3: GCS 14–13 and motor deficit
- Grade 4: GCS 12–7 with or without motor deficit
- Grade 5: GCS 6–3 with or without motor deficit

Other grading scales include Hunt and Hess, and the Fisher radiological scale.

8. What are the neurological complications that may be expected? [2 for all/1 for most]

There is a risk of rebleeding, with the greatest risk in the first 24 hours. The risk remains as high as 30% over the subsequent 4 weeks. Interventions are aimed at reducing this risk. There are two options: clipping and coiling. Clipping requires a craniotomy followed by the placement of clips around the neck of the aneurysm. Coiling is performed through femoral catheterization with platinum coils that obliterate the aneurysm by causing a blood clot to form in it.

There is also the risk of an intracerebral haematoma.

Hydrocephalus is another possible complication and an external ventricular drain may be needed.

Delayed cerebral ischaemia (DCI) – often caused by vasospasm – is a common complication. It peaks at 5 to 10 days and is attributed to the breakdown of blood products, release of inflammatory mediators, endothelial damage and microvascular thrombosis.

9. How would you diagnose vasospasm? [2 for all/1 for most]

There is a reduction in GCS in conscious patients with or without focal signs. Hypertensive surges, bradycardia, arrhythmias may also occur.

Cerebral angiography can be diagnostic and is the gold standard. CT/MR angiography or transcranial Doppler ultrasound scan are less invasive.

10. What are the options available to treat cerebral vasospasm? [3 for all/2 for most]

Available options include the following:

- Nimodipine
- Magnesium
- Endovascular treatments including balloon angioplasty + intra-arterial infusions of vasodilating agents
- Triple H therapy (hypervolaemia, hypertension and haemodilution) – although recent evidence seems to be against the use of hypervolaemia

Data 24

You are asked to assess a 70-year-old man who is day 9 post Ivor–Lewis oesophagectomy. His post-operative course was complicated by a hospital acquired pneumonia. He is now once again in respiratory distress and has a PaO_2 of 8.7 kPa on 15 litres via a non-rebreathe bag and is hypotensive and tachycardic with a blood pressure of 85/59 mmHg and heart rate of 110/min. He has a background history of hypertension and mild chronic obstructive pulmonary disease (COPD).

1. What is your immediate management? [2 for all, 1 for 2]

Check airway, breathing and circulation.
Carry out a fluid challenge.
Review notes and investigations.
Discuss and review the case with surgeons.
Arrange immediate transfer to critical care unit.

2. Would you use CPAP?

This requires discussion with the surgical team as swallowed air can put pressure on the anastomosis, especially if not decompressed with a nasogastric tube. High-flow nasal oxygen may be an acceptable alternative. If the patient requires respiratory support, this is usually invasive. [2]

3. This is his chest X-ray post intubation – comment on this.

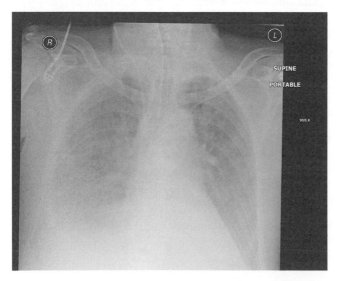

There is a portable anteroposterior film with an appropriately sited right internal jugular central venous catheter (RIJ CVC) and an endotracheal tube (ETT). There is volume loss on the right with widespread opacification. There is likely a pleural effusion on the right. [3]

4. What are your differential diagnoses?

This is a case of unresolved or new hospital acquired pneumonia. [1]

A pulmonary embolism is a possibility. [1]

An anastamotic leak could present in this way. [1]

5. This is a mid thoracic CT image following enteral contrast performed 2 days after intensive care admission. What does it demonstrate?

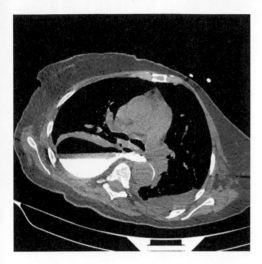

The CT shows bright white enteral contrast leaking from the distal oesophagus into a cavity in the right lower part of the thorax. There is non-contrast fluid in the cavity with a clear air–fluid interface. There is some consolidation around the cavity on the right and in the dependent left lung. [2]

6. How would you manage this complication? [4 for all]

You would manage either conservatively or surgically, balanced against the surgical view and the fitness of the patient.

Sometimes defunctioning of the oesophagus is required with a cervical oesophagostomy.

A conservative strategy could include keeping nil by mouth, intravenous antibiotics, total parenteral nutrition (TPN) and insertion of a large-bore intercostal drain in addition to other supportive care.

Upper gastro-intestinal secretions can be reduced by high-dose proton pump inhibitors and possibly octreotide.

7. The patient becomes agitated and pulls out their nasogastric tube. How should we manage this situation? [2 for both]

Discussion with the surgical team is key as blindly re-siting the tube risks further oesophageal damage or mediastinal placement.

A radiologically inserted NG tube over a wire is probably the safest option.

8. What options are there to prevent the NG tube being removed? [2 for both]

'Bridling' behind the nasal septum can fix the NG tube in position.

Attentive nursing care with reassurance, explanation and prevention and treatment of delirium should all help, but physical fixation may be needed.

Data 25

A 60-year-old man with a 2-month history of weight loss and abdominal distension presents feeling acutely unwell. His SpO_2 is 87% on air. This ECG has been done 30 minutes ago.

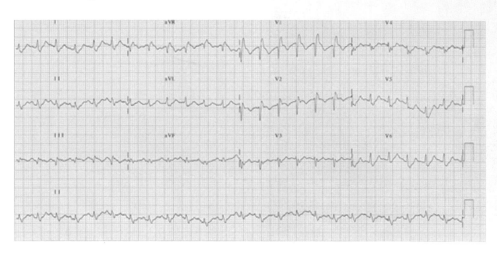

1. What does the ECG show?
It shows sinus tachycardia, right bundle branch block, T-wave inversion V1–3 and III. [2]

2. Give a differential diagnosis.   [2 for all]
- Pulmonary embolism (PE)
- Acute coronary syndrome
- Exclude pulmonary oedema, pneumonia and pneumothorax as causes for hypoxia

3. Suggest some suitable, immediate bedside investigations.   [2]
Include arterial blood gas tests, chest X-ray, serial ECGs, bedside echocardiography and blood tests such as troponin, D-dimer or brain natriuretic peptide (BNP/pro-BNP).   [2]

4. His chest X-ray is unremarkable. Name a scoring system appropriate to the likely diagnosis.   [2 for more than 1 system]
Several scoring systems are described, including the Wells score, Geneva score, the Pulmonary Embolism Severity Index (PESI) which can predict outcome once diagnosis of PE confirmed. The Pulmonary Embolism Rule-out Criteria (PERC) are used for ruling out low-probability cases.

5. What abnormal features might a transthoracic echocardiogram show that would support a diagnosis of pulmonary embolism?
Abnormal feautures include raised pulmonary artery (PA) pressures, right ventricular (RV) dilation, RV failure, McConnell's sign (a regional pattern of right ventricular dysfunction,

with akinesia of the mid free wall but normal motion at the apex) and direct visualization of thrombus in the PA (not very common). [2]

6. A CT pulmonary angiogram is performed. What does it show?

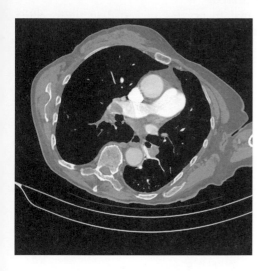

The PA trunk is opacified with contrast. There is a hypodense filling defect in the right proximal PA, which is a thrombus. [2]

7. Echocardiography shows severe RV dilatation. The patient's blood pressure is 115/65 mmHg and there are no signs of impaired peripheral perfusion. How would you categorize his clinical condition? [2 for both]

This is a 'sub-massive' PE. Definitions vary a bit, but generally this includes signs of RV dysfunction (which can be various), but without systemic shock/hypotension.

'Massive PE' means haemodynamic instability/hypotension/shock. (Previously this was defined anatomically by embolic size, > 50% obstruction of pulmonary vasculature).

8. What are the indications for thrombolysis?

There are various guidelines from the British Thoracic Society and the American Heart Association. Massive PE is defined as acute PE with sustained hypotension (systolic blood pressure < 90 mmHg for at least 15 minutes or requiring inotropic support, not due to a cause other than PE, such as arrhythmia, hypovolaemia, sepsis, or left ventricular (LV) dysfunction), pulselessness or persistent profound bradycardia (heart rate < 40 bpm with signs or symptoms of shock). Thrombolysis is indicated in massive PE.

In sub-massive PE the evidence is less certain. Some argue in favour of thrombolysis in relation to improving longer-term outcomes such as reducing the burden of RV failure or thrombus-related pulmonary hypertension; others point to the relatively low mortality rates even with standard treatment (heparin), and the known potential for serious morbidity/mortality of thrombolytics (mainly due to intracranial bleeding). [2]

9. What other treatments (apart from thrombolysis) should be considered?

Other treatments include the following: heparin (unfractionated or low-molecular-weight), an inferior vena cava filter, thrombectomy/interventional radiology procedures and longer-term anticoagulation (once diagnosis is confirmed). [2]

10. What other investigations should be considered?

Suitable investigations for likely underlying malignancy (as suggested in the opening question) should be considered, and possibly also a thrombophilia screen. [2]

Data 26

A 54-year-old lady has been admitted to the unit 5 days ago with severe sepsis secondary to cellulitis. She currently still requires multi-organ support with ventilation, vasopressors and renal replacement therapy. She remains on high-dose benzyl penicillin. Her sequential full blood count results are as follows.

	Day 1	Day 2	Day 3	Day 4	Day 5
Hb (g/dL)	11.1	9.2	8.4	7.9	7.2
WCC ($\times 10^9$/L)	19.2	16.4	11.4	13.3	15.1
Platelets ($\times 10^9$/L)	174	135	101	97	32
INR	1.3	1.3	1.1	1.2	1.2
APTT (27–35 seconds)	61	58	93	82	56

1. What are possible causes of this thrombocytopenia?
Thrombocytopenia can be classified into the following broad categories :
- Reduced production of platelets   [2 – if examples provided]
    . Bone marrow hypoplasia
    . Chronic alcoholism
    . Vitamin B12 deficiency
    . Drugs – methotrexate, valproate
    . Underlying haematological disease
- Increased sequestration of platelets   [2 – if examples provided]
    . Hypersplenism
- Increased destruction   [2 – if examples provided]
    . Immune mediated – ITP, SLE, drugs (penicillin, heparin)
    . Non-immune – TTP, DIC, HUS
    . Miscellaneous – sepsis, CVVH
    . Often multifactorial

2. This lady subsequently develops an axillary vein thrombosis – what diagnosis would you like to exclude?
She could have an inherited or acquired pro-thrombotic state, but with the blood results given, heparin-induced thrombocytopenia (HIT) should be excluded.   [2]

3. What is heparin, where is it produced and how does it work?
Heparin is a naturally occurring glycosaminoglycan.   [1]
It is produced by mast cells and basophils, derived from tissues rich in mast cells.   [1]
It increases antithrombin levels, which in turn inhibits thrombin and factor Xa.   [1]

4. What is the pathophysiology of HIT?

A slight fall in platelets of less than 30% occurs in up to a third of patients within 4 days of starting heparin – this is not HIT. HIT is seen more often with patients starting unfractionated heparin, typically occurring 5 to 10 days after starting treatment. It is less common with low-molecular-weight heparin (LMWH). [1]

Antibodies form against heparin and platelet factor 4 and together form a complex capable of activating and subsequently depleting platelets. [2]

5. How do you diagnose HIT?

Use the 4-T score (see below), which is based on the severity of thrombocytopenia, the timing of the fall in platelet count, the presence of thrombosis and whether or not other causes for thrombocytopenia exist. [1]

The diagnosis is confirmed by specific enzyme-linked immunosorbent assay (ELISA) tests but false positives and negatives are possible. Testing is usually therefore indicated in those with at least moderate probability of HIT from the 4-T scoring. [1]

6. How do you treat HIT?

Stop all heparin, including heparin within invasive line flush solutions. [1]

Substitute with other drugs. [2]

Use direct thrombin inhibitors, such as argatroban or factor Xa inhibitors, such as danaparoid or fondapurinux, at therapeutic doses.

Platelets transfusion is contraindicated; withhold warfarin until platelets have recovered (increased risk of thrombotic events). [1]

All treatment decisions should be discussed with a haematologist.

Further information

The following table gives details of the 4-T scoring system.

Feature	Score		
	2 points	1 point	0 points
Thrombocytopenia	> 50% fall and platelet nadir 20–100 × 10^9/L	30–50% fall or platelet nadir 10–19 × 10^9/L	> 30% fall or platelet nadir < 10 × 10^9/L
Timing of platelet count fall	Clear onset on day 5–10, or = 1 d if heparin exposure within past 30 d	Consistent with day 5–10 fall, but not clear (e.g., missing platelet counts); onset after day 10; or fall = 1 day if heparin exposure 30–100 days ago	Platelet count fall < 4 d without recent heparin exposure
Thrombosis or other sequelae	New thrombosis (confirmed); skin necrosis; acute systemic reaction after an intravenous unfractionated heparin bolus	Progressive or recurrent thrombosis; erythematous skin lesions; thrombosis suspected but not proven	None
Other causes of thrombocytopenia	None apparent	Possible	Definite

Total scores and corresponding probability of HIT are as follows:

- 0–3: Low probability
- 4–5: Intermediate probability
- 6–8: High probability

Data 27

You are asked to see a young man who is 7 days following a traumatic brain injury. His sedation has been off for 5 days and he hasn't woken up. He had a CT brain scan performed this morning.

1. **Tell me about the CT brain scan.**

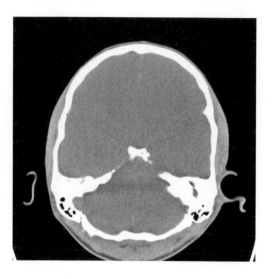

There is complete loss of grey–white matter differentiation affecting the whole of the brain, including the brainstem. This image is in keeping with brainstem death. [1]

2. **What are the criteria for brainstem death?** [2 for most]

Preconditions	Exclusions
Cause of coma known	No hypothermia
Irreversible	No sedative drugs
Patient deeply unconscious and requiring mechanical ventilation	No endocrine/metabolic disturbances
Adequate cardiovascular stability	No muscle relaxants

Reference: A code of practice for the diagnosis and confirmation of death. Academy of Medical Royal Colleges, 2008.

3. **Who can perform the testing?**
Brainstem tests are performed by at least two doctors who have been registered for more than 5 years and are competent in performing these tests. At least one of them should be a consultant. These individuals should have no clinical conflict of interest. Tests should be performed on two separate occasions. [2]

4. When is the legal time of death?

The legal time of death is the time of completion of the first set of tests confirming brainstem death. [1]

5. Describe the clinical tests for brainstem death and which cranial nerves are tested. [1 for each, max. 6]

1. Pupils are fixed and unresponsive to light – 2nd and 3rd cranial nerves.
2. There is no corneal reflex – 5th and 7th cranial nerves.
3. There is no oculo vestibular reflex: no eye movement to 50 mL ice-cold saline in each ear over 1 minute with clear tympanic membranes – 3rd , 6th and 8th cranial nerves.
4. There is no motor response to pain within cranial nerve distribution – 5th and 7th cranial nerves.
5. There are no gag or cough reflexes to stimulation – 9th and 10th cranial nerves.
6. There is apnoea to $PaCO_2 > 6.65kPa$ (confirmed with arterial blood gas).

6. Do we need to do any investigations to support the clinical diagnosis of brainstem death?

We do not usually have to perform any investigations. [1]

7. When might such tests be advisable? What is available? [3 for all]

Such tests would be advisable if there is concern regarding a high cervical cord injury, the apnoea test may be unreliable. Also, if other cranial nerve examinations cannot be performed, e.g. in the case of massive facial trauma.

Ancilliary tests may include four-vessel angiography, a transcranial Doppler scan, a PET scan, an ECG and an evoked potentials test.

8. Once a patient has been diagnosed as brainstem dead, is it reasonable or appropriate to insert a central line or start vasopressors to optimize the organs for the benefit of the recipient?

If organ donation is going to proceed, it is good practice to attempt to optimize organ function. [2]

9. What would you do if the patient was due to go to theatre in 2 hours for full retrieval of organs but suddenly went into ventricular fibrillation?

Most UK clinicians would see this as a step too far to resuscitate and make this clear to families when planning care of the donor. This is an interesting ethical question; there is no 'correct' answer but you need to justify whatever answer you give. [2]

Data 28

A 28-year-old lady with a history of severe depression is admitted to the emergency department with a suspected overdose. She is unconscious with a Glasgow Coma Score (GCS) of 3/15 and dilated but reactive pupils.

1. What does the ECG demonstrate?

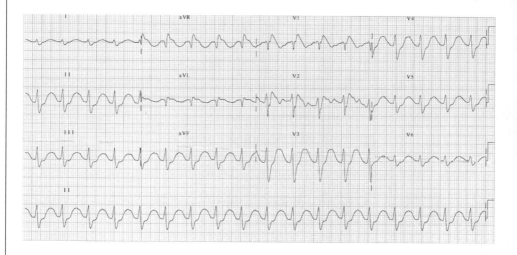

The ECG shows sinus tachycardia, a broad QRS complex, first-degree heart block and a borderline prolonged QTc interval.   [2]

2. This is the ECG 1 hour post admission. What does it demonstrate?

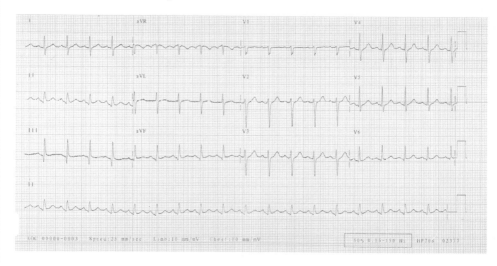

This ECG shows sinus tachycardia with a normal QRS complex. [2]

3. Which treatment is likely to have been given?

It is likely that this patient received sodium bicarbonate to treat a suspected tricyclic antidepressant (TCA) overdose. Other therapies to create a relative alkalosis could include hyperventilation if the patient was ventilated. [1]

4. What causes these ECG changes to develop?

A blockade of fast sodium channels results in a prolonged QRS complex and a predisposition to arrhythmias. Blockage of potassium channels can result in a prolonged QTc interval. [2]

5. What are the clinical features of a TCA overdose? [2 for all]

Classically, a TCA overdose presents with a mix of neurological and cardiac abnormalities (see *Emerg Med J*. 2011 Apr; 28(4): 347–368).

It can affect the central nervous system, causing seizures, convulsions and coma.

The cardiovascular system can also be affected, leading to sinus tachycardia, a prolonged QRS on the ECG, ventricular arrhythmias and hypotension.

6. How would you approach the management of this case?

Check airway, breathing and circulation, including intubation and ventilation. [1]

Consider gastric lavage if it is within 1 hour of presentation but protect the airway first with intubation. [1]

Use sodium bicarbonate to treat symptoms and signs of cardiotoxicity. Aim for a pH of 7.45–7.55 if dysrhythmia, hypotension or a widened QRS complex is present on the ECG. [1]

The use of magnesium may be considered for resistant arrhythmias. [1]

Other supportive therapies include the use of intravenous fluids and vasopressors to treat hypotension, and of benzodiazepines to manage seizures. [1]

Case reports suggest the potential role for lipid emulsions to treat life-threatening toxicity although evidence for this is limited. [1]

7. What is the mechanism of action of sodium bicarbonate?

Alkalinization primarily works through reducing the affinity of the drug to the sodium channel. [1]

8. Which drugs would you avoid using in this scenario?

In general, most antiarrhythmics drugs should be avoided as they can potentiate cardio toxicity. [1]

For example, quinidine, disopyramide (class 1a), phenytoin (class 1b) and flecainide (class 1c) can all potentiate a sodium-channel blockade. [1]

9. What does this ECG demonstrate?

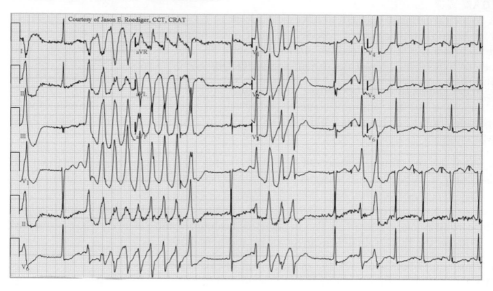

This ECG points to torsades de pointes, which is specific form of polymorphic ventricular tachycardia.   [2]

Data 29

A 40-year-old man with a history of hypertension presents with a 2-hour history of back pain radiating to the chest which came on whilst playing squash. The emergency department staff are concerned as he looks pale and clammy and ask for your advice.

1. What else do you want to know? [2 for most]

There are many causes of chest and back pain, but these can be considered as cardiac, lung, musculoskeletal or oesophago-gastric in origin. A hypertensive middle-aged man exerting himself is perhaps more likely to have had a cardiac problem. Key points would include:

- His history
  - Nature and characteristics of pain
  - Associated symptoms such as shortness of breath or palpitations
  - Past history/family history of cardiovascular problems
  - Risk factors for cardiac disease: smoking, hypertension, diabetes, hypercholesterolaemia
  - Drug use (cocaine or stimulants)
  - Medication history
- An examination
  - Standard cardiovascular, but look for Marfanoid features, neurology or peripheral hypoperfusion can indicate dissection
  - Tenderness may indicate muscular problems
  - Blood pressure in both arms
  - Murmurs of aortic incompetence, signs of tamponade
- Basic investigations
  - ECG to exclude cardiac event, CXR for lung pathology

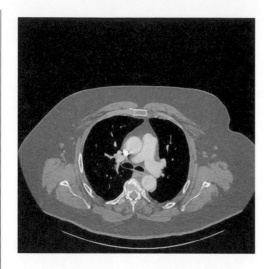

2. Tell me what you can see on this CT scan.

The image is a thoracic cross section taken at the level of the pulmonary trunk. Contrast has been given. There is an obvious dissection flap seen in the descending thoracic aorta with contrast in both the true and false lumens. [1]

There is no other gross pathology and no cardiac tamponade. [1]

3. What else do we need to see on the CT scan?

The proximal origin of the dissection flap is important, as this will guide treatment. [1]

The distal extent may give further cause for concern as the flap may involve the renal or mesenteric arteries or extend into the vessels perfusing the pelvis or limbs. [1]

There may be a haematoma, pleural effusion or cardiac tamponade. [1]

4. How do we classify dissections? [2 for all]

- The DeBakey system:
  - Type I – tear originates in ascending aorta and extends at least to the aortic arch or beyond
  - Type II – confined to the ascending aorta
  - Type III – originates in descending aorta
- Stanford classification:
  - A – involves the ascending aorta and/or aortic arch, and possibly the descending aorta
  - B – involves the descending aorta or the arch (distal to the left subclavian artery), without involvement of the ascending aorta

5. How do we typically treat these dissections? [1 for both]

Type A dissections often involve the aortic valve, which often becomes incompetent as a result. The valve will need re-seating and repair, which will also reduce the potential for coronary artery injury. The dissected thoracic aorta is usually replaced with a synthetic graft.

Mortality from type B dissections is better without surgery unless there is a distal associated perfusion problem, such as renal artery hypoperfusion. Complex endovascular proced-ures are increasingly common with standard or bespoke grafts.

6. The surgeons decide to treat without surgery and ask for your help. How would you treat this man conservatively?

The key is blood-pressure control. This will need invasive arterial monitoring and usually infusions of titratable antihypertensive medications. [1]

The target mean arterial pressure is usually 60–75 mmHg (or the lowest blood pressure tolerated). [1]

Assess perfusion indices such as lactate, base deficit, urine output and neurology regularly. [1]

Analgesia and anxiolysis are important in controlling BP. [1]

Negative inotropes may be required to reduce the force of blood ejected from the left ventricle, used in combination with vasodilators. [1]

7. What drugs would you use? [2 for all]

Beta blockers are the first line of treatment and rapidly acting, titratable parenteral agents such as esmolol or labetalol are suitable.

Calcium channel blockers can be used if beta blockers are contraindicated. Verapamil and diltiazem are ideal as they are negatively inotropic and chronotropic.

Vasodilators such as sodium nitroprusside or GTN can be used but these may cause reflex tachycardias if used alone.

8. What if the patient remains hypertensive despite using these three classes of drug?

You should address his pain and anxiety. [1]

Consider using centrally acting drugs such as clonidine. [1]

Consider an extension of the dissection to involve renal vessels. [1]

Data 30

A 74-year-old man has just undergone elective angiography to investigate myocardial ischaemia. Endovascular approach was via the femoral artery. He develops tachycardia and hypotension and is described as pale. He has had a previous myocardial infarction which resulted in poor left-ventricular function and he has a history of hypertension.

Initial blood results are below.

		Reference range
Sodium	140 mmol/L	136–145 mmol/L
Potassium	4.8 mmol/L	3.6–5.2 mmol/L
Urea	10 mmol/L	2.5–6.4 mmol/L
Creatinine	130 µmol/L	80–132 µmol/L
WCC	14.2×10^9/L	$4–11 \times 10^9$/L
Haemoglobin	6.7 g/dL	11.5–16.5 g/dL
Platelets	220×10^9/L	$150–400 \times 10^9$/L
INR	1.2	

1. How would you assess and manage this patient?

This man has significant shock, which is likely a combination of cardiogenic or hypovolaemic components. There may be major bleeding. Management will include the following: [3 for all, 2 for most]

- Check airway, breathing, circulation, disability and exposure (ABCDE approach) including the administration of 15 litres O_2 via non-rebreather mask (titrated oxygen therapy)
- Obtain large-bore intravenous access and ensuring blood for cross-match
- Give O negative or cross-matched blood depending on the urgency of the situation
- Check arterial blood gas, full blood count, urea and electrolytes and clotting
- Electrocardigram (ECG) and/or bedside echocardiogram (tamponade or new ischaemia is a possibility)
- Targeted inotropic support may be indicated.
- Urinary catheterization

2. **He develops respiratory failure and he is intubated and ventilated. This is his chest X-ray. Briefly, what does it show and what are the likely causes?**

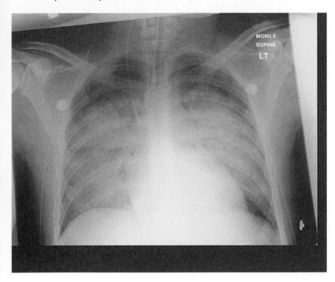

This is a mobile supine chest X-ray of an intubated patient with a right internal jugular central venous catheter (RIJ CVC) and ECG monitoring. Allowing for projection, the heart size appears normal. There is extensive bilateral shadowing in both lung fields, mostly mid and lower zones that is more dense centrally, with a few air bronchograms visible. [1]

Features are consistent with pulmonary oedema, likely secondary to left ventricular failure given the history. [1]

Another possibility is acute respiratory distress syndrome (ARDS) which could be due to a primary cause (pneumonia) or secondary (organ ischaemia). [1]

3. **He is noted to have increasing abdominal distension 6 hours later on the intensive care unit and the nurses tell you his abdomen is very tense. How would you assess this?**

You should perform a detailed clinical assessment – including an abdominal examination, looking out for bruising, tenderness and guarding. [1]

Further investigations include CT of the abdomen if the patient is stable enough. A bedside FAST (focused assessment with sonography in trauma) scan may provide useful diagnostic information in the haemodynamically unstable patient. [1]

Measure the intra-abdominal pressure via urinary catheter. [1]

4. **His oxygenation is getting worse and his $PaCO_2$ on the blood gas is rising. Can you explain what might be happening to cause this?**

Assuming the ventilator settings have not been reduced, a reduction in minute volume is likely to have occurred as the thoracic compliance decreases, reflecting the likely intra-abdominal hypertension. [1]

5. **Subsequently, his renal function is found to be: urea 15 mmol/L, creatinine 300 μmol/L. What are the likely causes?** [1 for each category with example, max. 3]

Likely causes of worsening acute kidney injury in this scenario include:

- *Pre-renal* – acute kidney injury secondary to shock (hypovolaemia + poor cardiac function); intra-abdominal hypertension can compromise renal blood supply and venous drainage
- *Renal* – as a result of contrast used during angiography or CT scans; direct pressure effects from a retro-peritoneal haemorrhage
- *Post-renal* – less likely but ensure patient is catheterized and review imaging to exclude intra-renal and post-renal obstruction

6. **Can you define intra-abdominal hypertension (IAH) and abdominal compartment syndrome (ACS)?** [2 for all]

ACS is defined as a sustained intra-abdominal pressure (IAP) > 20 mmHg (with or without an abdominal perfusion pressure (APP) < 60 mmHg) that is associated with new organ dysfunction/failure. (Note that the normal IAP is approximately 5–7 mmHg in critically ill adults, and APP = MAP – IAP.)

IAH is defined by a sustained or repeated pathologic elevation of IAP $\geq$ 12 mmHg.

IAH is graded as follows: Grade I: IAP 12–15 mmHg, Grade II: IAP 16–20 mmHg, Grade III: IAP 21–25 mmHg, Grade IV: IAP > 25 mmHg.

Primary ACS is a condition associated with injury or disease in the abdomino-pelvic region that frequently requires early surgical or radiological intervention.

Secondary ACS refers to conditions that do not originate from the abdomino-pelvic region.

7. **Describe the measurement of intra-abdominal pressure** [2 for all]

Direct measurement of IAP is carried out by means of an intra-peritoneal catheter, or indirectly by transduction of pressures from the indwelling femoral vein or the use of rectal, gastric or urinary bladder catheters.

A Foley catheter may be used. Sterile saline (50–100 mL is described, but the standard is now 25 mL) is injected into the empty bladder through the catheter. The sterile tubing of the urinary drainage bag is cross-clamped just distal to the culture aspiration port. The end of the drainage bag tubing is then connected to the catheter. The clamp is released just enough to allow the tubing proximal to the clamp to flow fluid from the bladder, and then reapplied. A 16-gauge needle is then used to Y-connect a manometer or pressure transducer through the culture aspiration port of the tubing of the drainage bag. Finally, the top of the symphysis pubic bone is used as the zero point with the patient supine.

An alternative bedside technique has been described in which intragastric pressure measurements are taken from an indwelling nasogastric tube. This method has been validated and found to vary within 2.5 cmH$_2$O of urinary bladder pressures.

8. **What are the principles of management of intra-abdominal hypertension?**
[3 for all, 2 for most]

1. Conservative management:
   - Minimization of intra-luminal contents
   - Evacuation of any space-occupying lesions (clots, abscesses)

- Relaxed abdominal wall (sedate, paralyse)
- Not too much fluid
- Optimization of the perfusion of viscera
- Active prevention – non-primary closure of high-risk abdomens
2. Surgical management:
   - Decompression (laparostomy)

Data 31

A 45-year-old male poly-trauma patient has been admitted to a local intensive care unit. This is a section of the drug chart. These drugs were given in this specific combination for prophylactic effect.

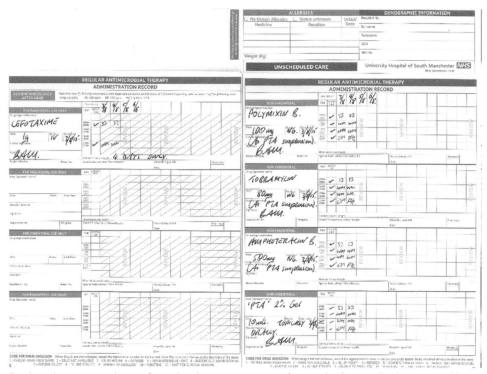

For the colour version, please refer to the plate section. In some formats this figure will only appear in black and white.

1. What could this combination of drugs represent?
This combination of drugs indicates therapy targeted towards a selective decontamination of the digestive tract (SDD). [1]

2. What is the goal of SDD?
The goal of SDD is to prevent, or to eradicate (if initially present) oropharyngeal and gastro-intestinal carriage of potentially pathogenic microorganisms (PPMs). SDD is active against community or hospital acquired PPM but is thought to preserve non-pathological indigenous flora, which in turn are thought to protect against overgrowth with antibiotic-resistant bacteria. [1]

3. What are the classic components of SDD? [1 for principles, 2 for all]
SDD classically consists of four aspects:
1. Selective eradication of PPMs in the oral cavity by application of orabase, containing non-absorbable antibiotics (e.g. polymyxin B, tobramycin and amphotericin B – often

called 'PTA'), and decontamination of the rest of the digestive tract by local administration (through a nasogastric tube) of these antibiotics.
2. Systemic prophylaxis (e.g. cefotaxime) to prevent respiratory infections that may occur early during the intensive care unit stay, caused by commensal respiratory flora (*Streptococcus pneumoniae* and *Haemophilus influenzae*).
3. Ensuring optimal hygiene, to prevent cross-contamination.
4. Regular cultures of throat swabs and faeces are performed (monitoring the effectiveness of SDD).

4. What are the potential benefits of SDD [1 for overview, 2 if specific]
The aim is to reduce the risks of nosocomial infections.
The majority of primary intensive care unit infections are caused by opportunistic aerobic Gram-negative bacilli (*Klebsiella, Proteus, Morganella, Enterobacter, Citrobacter, Serratia, Acinetobacter* and *Pseudomonas)* that are present in individuals with underlying pathology and are proceeded by colonization of the gastro-intestinal tract in many cases.

5. What problems can result from SDD?
The biggest concern is about antibiotic resistance, but also diarrhoea. [1]

6. What is a nosocomial infection?
This is an infection acquired in hospital by a patient who was admitted for a reason other than that infection. It is an infection occurring in a patient in a hospital or other healthcare facility in whom the infection was not present or incubating at the time of admission. This includes infections acquired in the hospital but appearing after discharge, and also occupational infections among staff of the facility. [1]

7. What is the time 'cut-off' for this definition?
Historically, this is given at 48 hours but this doesn't make allowances for the patient's carrier status and has been questioned. Up to 3 days after discharge or up to 30 days after an operation are also commonly used definitions. [1]

8. Can you give me some examples? [1 for 2 or more]
Urinary-tract infections are the most common type of nosocomial infection. Surgical site infections, bloodstream infections, and pneumonia are the other most common types (according to the WHO, 2012). Particular emphasis is currently placed on infections caused by methicillin-resistant *Staphylococcus aureus* (MRSA), vancomycin-resistant enterococci (VRE) and *Clostridium difficile*.

9. What is *Clostridium difficile*?
It is a Gram-positive spore-forming bacteria that is best known for causing antibiotic-associated diarrhoea. While it can be a normal component of colonic flora, the bacterium is thought to cause disease when competing bacteria in the gut have been wiped out by antibiotic treatment. It is the most common cause of pseudomembranous colitis and in rare cases this can progress to toxic megacolon, which is a life-threatening complication. [1]

10. What are the risk factors for *Clostridium difficile* infection (CDI)? [1 for all]
There is a risk from exposure to broad-spectrum antibiotics.
There is increasing evidence that acid-suppressing medications, in particular proton pump inhibitors (PPIs), may be a risk factor.
Poor infection prevention practices also play a major role in its spread.

11. How do you assess the severity of *Clostridium Difficile* infection (CDI)? [1 for classification, 2 for detail]

Mild CDI is not associated with a raised white cell count (WCC); it is typically associated with < 3 stools of type 5–7 on the Bristol Stool Chart per day.

Moderate CDI is associated with a raised WCC that is < 15 10^9/L; it is typically associated with 3–5 stools per day.

Severe CDI is associated with a WCC > 15 10^9/L, or an acute rising serum creatinine (i.e. > 50% increase above baseline), or a temperature of > 38.5 °C or evidence of severe colitis (abdominal or radiological signs). The number of stools may be a less reliable indicator of severity.

Life-threatening CDI includes hypotension, partial or complete ileus or toxic megacolon, or CT evidence of severe disease.

12. How do you treat CDI?

Supportive care should be given, including attention to hydration, electrolytes and nutrition. Antiperistaltic agents should be avoided in acute infection. [1]

The precipitating antibiotic should be stopped wherever possible; agents with less risk of inducing CDI can be substituted if an underlying infection still requires treatment. [1]

For *mild* and *moderate* CDI, give oral metronidazole for 10–14 days. [1]

For *severe* CDI, give oral vancomycin 10–14 days. Refractory cases can be treated with a combination of high-dose oral vancomycin plus intravenous metronidazole or fidaxomicin (see the 'Updated guidance on the management and treatment of *Clostridium difficile* infection' by Public Health England). The addition of oral rifampicin or intravenous immunoglobulin may also be considered. [1]

Patients with severe CDI should have specialist surgical input, and should have their blood lactate measured. Colectomy should be considered, especially if caecal dilatation is > 10 cm. Colectomy is best performed before blood lactate rises > 5 mmol/L, when survival is extremely poor. [1]

Data 32

A 55-year-old woman received a haemopoetic stem cell transplant (HSCT) for acute myeloid leukaemia. She presents 4 weeks after her transplant complaining of a dry cough, fevers and dyspnoea. This is her chest X-ray, and the following blood tests are obtained.

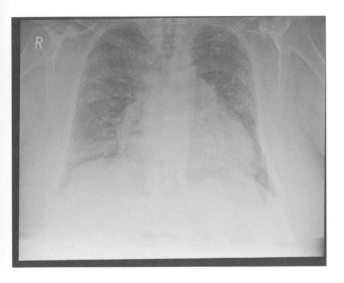

		Reference range
Sodium	136 mmol/L	136–145 mmol/L
Potassium	4.5 mmol/L	3.6–5.2 mmol/L
Urea	15 mmol/L	2.5–6.4 mmol/L
Creatinine	193 µmol/L	80–132 µmol/L
WCC	7.8×10^9/L	$4–11 \times 10^9$/L
Neutrophils	6.8×10^9/L	$2–7.5 \times 10^9$/L
Haemoglobin	9.7 g/dL	11.5–16.5 g/dL
Platelets	54×10^9/L	$150–400 \times 10^9$/L
Albumin	24 g/L	35–50 g/L
Total bilirubin	53 µmol/L	3–17 µmol/L
Alkaline phosphatase	98 IU/L	50–136 IU/L
ALT	145 IU/L	30–65 IU/L

1. What does the chest radiograph show?

It shows diffuse bilateral ground glass shadowing with air bronchograms in keeping with alveolar infiltration. [1]

2. What are the causes of this appearance?

There are a wide range of differentials so the answer should be structured: infective or non-infective.

- Infective causes: pneumonia (bacterial, viral or fungal) [1 mark for all 3]
- Non-infective causes, including the following: [1 for 2, 2 for all]
  - Cardiogenic pulmonary oedema (cardiac failure may be a consequence of chemotherapy prior to stem cell transplant)
  - Idiopathic pneumonia syndrome (diffuse lung injury with no infective cause)
  - Diffuse alveolar haemorrhage
  - Bronchiolitis obliterans organizing pneumonia (pulmonary complication thought to be related to graft versus host disease)

3. How would you investigate this lady on the basis of the chest X-ray findings?

You should run the following investigations:

- Culture infective agents: [2]
  - Send blood, sputum and ideally broncho-alveolar lavage (BAL) for M/C/S
  - Throat swabs, BAL for respiratory viral screen and viral load (adenovirus, rhinovirus, Epstein–Barr virus (EBV), influenza and parainfluenza, respiratory syncytial virus (RSV), herpes simplex virus (HSV) and cytomegalovirus (CMV))
  - Atypical serology
  - Aspergillus culture/galactomannan/polymerase chain reaction (PCR)

- *Pneumocystis jirovecii pneumonia* ('PJP', more commonly known as 'PCP') PCR from induced sputum/BAL
- Confirm/exclude cardiogenic cause: [1]
  - 12-lead electrocardiography
  - Transthoracic echocardiography
- Consider high-resolution CT of the chest [1]

4. Describe the abnormalities present in her blood tests [1 for 2, 2 for all]

A number of abnormalities are present:
- Anaemia
- Thrombocytopenia
- Hyperbilirubinaemia with elevated ALT
- Deranged urea and creatinine (may reflect acute kidney injury but requires correlation with old results)

5. What are the potential causes of the deranged liver function tests (LFTs)? [2]

- Sepsis
- Drug-related (antiviral/antifungal/antibiotic prophylaxis)
- Viral (e.g. EBV) or fungal infection
- Graft versus host disease (a triad of hepatitis/dermatitis/enteritis)
- Veno-occlusive disease (thrombosis of small hepatic venules following high-dose chemotherapy)
- Congestive cardiac failure leading to hepatic engorgement (chemotherapy preconditioning can lead to impaired left ventricular function)

6. Why does she have low platelets?

Thrombocytopenia is the commonest coagulopathy seen in haematological malignancy. This could be due to:
- Reduced survival of platelets in the circulation secondary to [2 for most]
  - Sepsis
  - Graft versus host disease
  - Veno-occlusive disease
  - Heparin-induced thrombocytopenia
  - Thrombotic thrombocytopenic purpura (TTP) – can occur after transplant
- Decreased production of platelets (poorly functioning graft), which occurs for the following reasons: [2 for most]
  - Insufficient transplanted cells
  - Weak bone marrow further impaired by infection/drugs
  - Marrow fibrosis
  - Graft versus host effect
  - Recurrence/persistence of the original malignancy

7. How can a haemopoetic stem cell transplant be classified? [2 marks for any three, 1 mark for two]

a. A haemopoetic stem cell transplant can be classified according to the source of the donor:
  - Autologous (the patient's own cells)
  - Allogenic (from a donor).

b. The classification depends on whether the donated cells are matched (to human leuco-cyte antigens) or unmatched.

c. It depends on the source of the cells, which are either peripheral, from the bone marrow or from cord blood.

d. Classification is also dependent on the intensity of the pre-transplant chemotherapy regime:
  - Myeloablative (total destruction of the patient's native bone marrow)
  - Reduced intensity conditioning (partial destruction of native bone marrow, tumour cells subsequently destroyed by donor cells).

8. What features would imply a poor prognosis for this lady?   [2 for all]
- Multi-organ failure
- Need for mechanical ventilation
- Need for renal replacement therapy
- Acute graft versus host disease
- Relapse of underlying malignancy after HSCT

Comment

Between 10 and 40% of patients require critical care following bone marrow transplantation (a lay term used to describe HSCT). Prognosis is often poor but improvements in critical care (e.g. prompt admission and use of non-invasive ventilation) along with better patient selection have led to falling mortality rates. The recipients of a bone marrow transplant have a weakened physiological reserve prior to critical care admission as a consequence of 'pre-conditioning' with chemotherapy/radiotherapy prior to transplant. The complications of bone marrow transplant are multi-system and are broadly due to complications of pre-conditioning, immunosuppression or graft versus host disease. Sepsis should always be suspected and the presentation may be non-specific as a consequence of impaired immune response.

Data 33

You are called to review a 64-year-old male in the emergency department, who has been admitted with a 1-week history of progressive lethargy and worsening dyspnoea following an upper respiratory infection. The patient is confused so the history has been obtained from his wife. Over the last few days he has not eaten and been unable to get out of bed. He has no significant past medical history and is on no medication. Initial observations are below:

Observation	Value
SpO$_2$ (FiO$_2$ 0.6)	93%
Respiratory rate	32 breaths/min
Heart rate	116 beats/min
Blood pressure	170/100 mmHg
Temperature	37.5 °C

He was catheterized shortly after admission, but has passed no urine after 2 hours. His initial blood results and arterial blood gas results are shown below:

		Reference range
Sodium	136 mmol/L	136–145 mmol/L
Potassium	7.1 mmol/L	3.6–5.2 mmol/L
Urea	54.3 mmol/L	2.5–6.4 mmol/L
Creatinine	826 µmol/L	80–132 µmol/L
Creatinine (2 months ago)	102 µmol/L	
C reactive protein	54 mg/L	< 3.0 mg/L
WCC	12.2 × 10^9/L	4–11 × 10^9/L
Haemoglobin	110 g/L	11.5–16.5 g/L
Platelets	164 × 10^9/L	150–400 × 10^9/L
pH	7.15	7.35–7.45
pO$_2$	8.3 kPa	10.0–14 kPa
pCO$_2$	3.3 kPa	4.4–5.9 kPa
Lactate	2.4 mmol/L	0–2 mmol/L
Base excess	−12	−2–(+2)

1. **Based on the limited information available to you, what are your key concerns at this stage?**
- Acute kidney injury (AKI)
  i. Severe hyperkalaemia [2]
  ii. Metabolic acidosis
- Hypoxia
- Hypertension

2. **Can you classify the causes of AKI?** [3 for all, 2 for most with structure, 1 for structure only]

- *Pre-renal (renal hypoperfusion)*:
  . Shock: distributive, obstructive, cardiogenic, hypovolaemic
  . Drugs: angiotensin-converting enzyme (ACE) or angiotensin II inhibitors, non-steroidal anti-inflammatory drugs (NSAIDs)
  . Hepatorenal syndrome
- *Intrinsic renal*:
  . Acute tubular necrosis
    – Ischaemia – prolonged hypoperfusion
    – Nephrotoxins
      a. Exogenous
        ▪ Drugs (e.g. aminoglycosides, amphotericin b, acyclovir)
        ▪ Ethylene glycol
        ▪ Radiological contrast
      b. Endogenous
        ▪ Uric acid (acute uric acid nephropathy)
        ▪ Myoglobin (rhabdomyolysis)
        ▪ Haemoglobin (haemolysis)
        ▪ Light chains (myeloma)
  . Vascular
    – Large vessel (renal artery/vein stenosis)
    – Small vessel (vasculitis/haemolytic uraemic syndrome (HUS)/thrombotic thrombocytopenic purpura (TTP)/malignant hypertension/scleroderma)
  . Glomerular disease
    – IgA glomerulonephritis
    – Goodpasture's syndrome
    – Acute post-infectious glomerulonephritis
    – Lupus nephritis
    – Granulomatosis polyangitis (Wegeners)
  . Acute interstitial nephritis
    – Drugs (e.g. penicillins, cephalosporins, furosemide, phenytoin, NSAIDs)
    – Infection (e.g. streptococcal, staphylococcal, legionella, Epstein–Barr virus (EBV), tuberculosis)
- *Post-renal*:
  . Obstruction within renal tract (urethral, bladder, ureteric)

3. How can we classify the severity of acute kidney injury?

One recognized approach is to use the KDIGO staging system for AKI (Kidney Disease: Improving Global Outcomes (KDIGO) Acute Kidney Injury Work Group. (*Kidney Int.*, 2012, Suppl. 2: 1–138.) [2]

Stage	Creatinine	Urine output
1	1.5–1.9 × baseline (known or presumed to have occurred within the last 7 days) *or* Increase ≥ 26.5 μmol/L above baseline (within 48 hours)	< 0.5 mL/kg per hour for 6–12 hours
2	2–2.9 × baseline	< 0.5 mL/kg per hour for ≥ 12 hours
3	≥ 3 × baseline *or* increase in creatinine to ≥ 353.6 μmol/L (must meet stage 1 criteria) *or* initiation of renal replacement therapy (RRT)	< 0.3mL/kg per hour for ≥ 24 hours *or* anuria ≥ 12 hours

4. How would you investigate this patient further?

- Blood tests [2 for most]
  - Blood cultures
  - Immune screen (ANA, anti-dsDNA, ANCA, C3/C4, anti-glomerular basement membrane antibodies, anti-streptolysin O titre (ASOT))
  - Uric acid
  - Creatine kinase
  - Myeloma screen (serum protein electrophoresis, serum free light chains)
  - Calcium/phosphate
- Imaging
  - Chest X-ray [2 for both]
  - Ultrasound of the renal tract – rule out obstructive cause of AKI
- Electrocardiogram (hyperkalaemia) [1]
- Urine (dipstick, MC+S (microscopy, culture and sensitivities), urine electrophoresis (myeloma) [1]

5. This is his chest X-ray. What does it show?

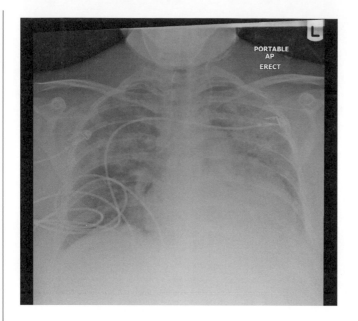

Portable, AP erect film. ECG monitoring *in situ* and a left internal jugular central line is appropriately placed. Even allowing for the AP projection, the heart appears enlarged. There are marked bilateral pulmonary infiltrates with no obvious focal consolidation. [1]

6. The patient subsequently starts coughing up fresh blood. What are the likely differentials?

This man has a likely pulmonary renal syndrome. The causes of this include: [2]

- Goodpasture's syndrome
- Vasculitis – Wegener's granulamatosis, polyarteritis
- Systemic lupus erythematosus (SLE)

7. The immunologist calls you to tell you that this man has a strongly positive anti-glomerular basement membrane antibody titres. How would you confirm your diagnosis? What specific treatment would you consider instituting?

Goodpasture's syndrome is the likely diagnosis and a renal biopsy would confirm this. [1]

Treatment would include treating hyperkalaemia and the patient is likely to need renal replacement therapy. [1]

Specific treatment for Goodpasture's would include immunosuppressants such as cyclophosphamide, steroids and plasmapheresis to aid clearance of auto-antibodies. [2]

Data 34

An 18-year-old man is brought to your emergency department following a high-speed motorbike accident where he hit a tree chest-on. He is awake and complaining of chest pain when he arrives and you are asked to see him following a chest X-ray. A primary survey does not raise any concerns of other significant injuries.

1. Please comment on his chest X-ray below.

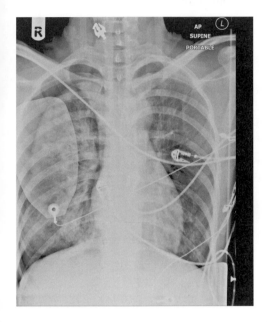

This is an anteroposterior supine, portable film of adequate penetration and exposure. Electrocardiogram monitoring and hands-free defibrillating pads are on the chest wall, partially obscuring a significant right-sided pneumothorax. There is a smaller left-sided pneumothorax seen too. Of note, there is no mediastinal air and the heart is central. There is no obvious gas under the diaphragm in this trauma patient.   [2]

2. What factors would make you consider intubating this trauma patient?   [3 for all]
He has a significant chest injury and gas exchange is likely to get worse, acutely or due to subsequent acute lung injury or contusion.
You should consider intubation if there is any suggestion of head injury or indication for CT scanning.
You should also consider intubation if there are any injuries that are going to need imminent surgical intervention.

3. He becomes increasingly hypoxic and needs intubation. What do you need to consider in planning intubation?   [4 for all]
You should consider cardiovascular stability – is he adequately resuscitated to tolerate induction?

He is at high risk of cervical spine injury and so appropriate in-line immobilization measures should be undertaken.

He is also at significant risk of a head injury and so a 'neuroprotective' induction with an opiod and agents to maintain arterial blood pressure should be used.

His chest injuries mean that he is at high risk of rapidly developing tension pneumothoraces as soon as positive pressure ventilation is commenced.

4. Would you insert chest drains before induction?

He will need bilateral intercostal drains at some point but it can be difficult to site surgical drains in an agitated patient who is in pain. If the clinical condition allows bilateral drains to be inserted prior to induction then this is probably the safest course of action. If the patient is unstable, decompressing the chest with temporary intercostal needles followed by immediate chest drains after securing the airway could be argued. [2]

5. Following induction and chest drainage, he becomes haemodynamically unstable. What should you do? [2 for both]

Haemorrhage should be excluded. Clinical examination and appropriate imaging (FAST ultrasound scanning or CT) should be undertaken.

Obstructive causes of shock such as tamponade or tension pneumothoraces should be considered, along with aortic dissection (from the mechanism of injury).

6. He is transferred to theatre for a laparotomy. This is his chest X-ray after the procedure. What has happened in theatre?

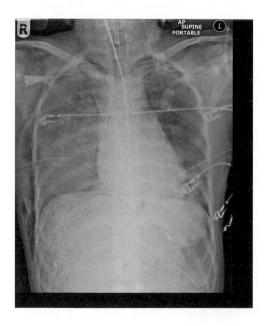

The chest X-ray clearly shows a large surgical pack under the right hemidiaphragm, extending across the midline. Whilst this could be a retained swab, it is likely that he has undergone damage control laparotomy with packing of the liver. [1]

7. What else can you see on his X-ray?   [1 for pneumothorax, 1 for at least 4 others]
- Residual right-sided pneumothorax
- Bilateral intercostal drains (in appropriate positions)
- Endotracheal tube
- Oesophageal Doppler probe
- Right subclavian and left internal jugular central lines
- Air under the left hemidiaphragm
- Subcutaneous emphysema, especially on the right flank

8. What should we do about the persistent pneumothorax?
There is evidence of a pneumothorax despite an adequately sited chest drain. The management of this would include seeking cardiothoracic opinion, inserting a second chest drain or application of low grade suction to the existing drain (which could increase air leak and reduce minute ventilation).   [1]

9. On day 3, his chest drain bubbling resumes and continues unhindered over the next 24 hours. What do you think may have caused this to happen?
Broncho-pleural fistula is a possibility that needs considering given the circumstances. [1]

10. How would you manage a broncho-pleural fistula in a ventilated patient?   [2 for all]
The ventilatory management is challenging and includes low tidal volume ventilation, minimizing airway pressures, and using low positive end expiratory pressure (PEEP) strategies.
A transition to a spontaneous mode of ventilation may be beneficial in aiding the weaning of respiratory support.
Other techniques described include the use of independent lung ventilation using double lumen tubes, even with two ventilators.
Suction applied to the chest drain can also help.

Data 35

A 48-year-old man is referred for consideration of critical care admission. He has a history of myasthenia gravis (MG) and has been admitted with a suspected lower respiratory tract infection. You are asked to assess the patient and determine whether he requires admission to the critical care unit for respiratory support. He is conscious and alert with a respiratory rate of 24 per minute, oxygen saturation of 94% on 8 litres oxygen and stable haemodynamic parameters. His chest X-ray shows no obvious focal pathology.

1. What is this test and what does it show?

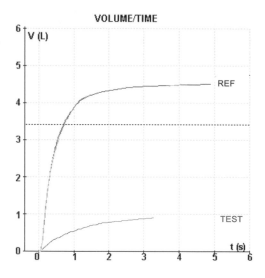

This is a vitalograph measurement showing a poor expiratory effort, reduced FEV1, reduced expiratory time and FVC of < 1 litre. [2]

2. **What features would suggest that this patient requires admission?**
Specific reasons for admission in this case could include:
- Respiratory failure – type 1 or type 2 secondary to his infection or a myasthenic crisis [1]
- Bulbar palsy and risk of aspiration [1]
- Vital capacity < 15mL/kg [1]

3. **Describe the pathophysiology of the condition.** [3 for all]
MG is an autoimmune condition characterized by the presence of autoantibodies against the post-synaptic nicotinic acetylcholine receptor (AChR) at the neuromuscular junction. It commonly affects young females and older males and is often associated with the presence of a thymoma.
Characteristic features include muscle weakness, fatiguability and ptosis. Respiratory, ocular and bulbar muscles are frequently involved.

4. How is it diagnosed? [1 each for clinical signs, antibodies and tensilon test]

Clinical suspicion based on the history and demonstrating muscle fatiguability should lead to testing with serum AChR autoantibodies.

Anti-AChR antibodies are present in 80% of cases, and are diagnostic of MG if present.

Anti-MuSK (muscle-specific receptor tyrosine kinase) antibodies are present in 70% of cases where Anti-AChR antibodies are absent.

If electromyography (EMG) is carried out, a greater than 10% decrement is demonstrated on repeated compound motor action potentials.

An edrophonium (tensilon) test can be helpful – there is a rapid improvement of symptoms following intravenous injection of edrophonium (a short-acting anticholinesterase).

5. What is a myasthenic crisis? What triggers it? [3 for all, 2 for most]

This is a severe and acute form of the disease resulting in the requirement for ventilatory support. It can be triggered by various factors including:

- Infection
- Pulmonary aspiration
- Trauma and surgery
- Stress
- Pregnancy
- Change in normal medication
- Drugs, including antibiotics such as gentamicin and ciprofloxacin that interact with the neuromuscular junction or beta blockers and magnesium that can affect action potentials

6. You measure the patient's vital capacity and it is 700 mL. The patient is admitted to the critical care unit for ongoing treatment. Describe your immediate management.

Check airway, breathing and circulation and the arterial blood gas analysis. [1]

Closely monitor respiratory status and muscle strength including regular forced vital capacity (FVC) measurements. [1]

A trial of non-invasive ventilation could be considered with escalation to intubation and invasive ventilation if required. It is important to note that these patients exhibit an unpredictable response to depolarizing muscle relaxants and are very sensitive to the action of non-depolarizing muscle relaxants. [1]

Plasma exchange or intravenous immunoglobulin, which is as effective as plasma exchange and often simpler to administer, may be considered. [1]

7. The patient recovers and is planned to be discharged to the ward. What maintenance treatment will you commence before discharge?

The mainstays of treatment are anticholinesterase therapy (usually the long acting pyridostigmine) and maintenance of immunosuppression (usually oral steroids and/or azathioprine). [2]

Data 36

A 44-year-old fit and well smoker attends accident and emergency with severe back pain of sudden onset whilst playing football. He is hypotensive. His ECG is shown below:

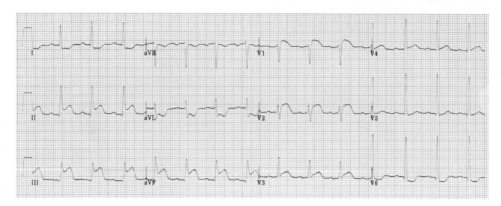

1. From the history alone, what is your differential diagnosis?
This could be an upper gastro-intestinal perforation or ulcer, pneumothorax, cardiac ischaemia or pericarditis, aortic dissection or a pulmonary embolism.   [1 for 4 or more]

2. Talk me through the ECG.
It shows a sinus rhythm, 100 beats per minute approximately, with a normal axis. There is ST elevation in the inferior leads. The ST elevation is more marked in III (which is more rightward facing) than II. There is also ST elevation in V1 and V2. This suggests an acute inferior wall myocardial infarction and associated right ventricular (RV) infarction.   [1]

3. Are there any other ECG techniques you can use to help diagnosis?
You could do a right-sided ECG.   [1]

4. What does this ECG show?

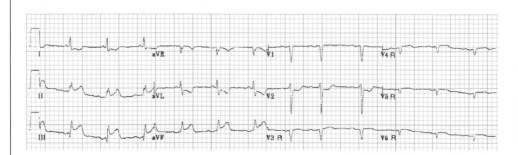

This shows ST elevation in the right-sided leads (V3R–V6R). [1]

5. What treatment would you institute?

Suitable treatments include administering O_2, antiplatelet agents and morphine. Nitrates can cause hypotension in RV infarcts. [1]

Consider thrombolysis versus percutaneous coronary intervention (PCI). [1]

6. What would an echocardiogram likely show?

It may show a dilated, non-contracting right ventricle. [1]

7. What would the central venous pressure read? Why?

It would be high. A poorly functioning right ventricle leads to elevated venous 'back' pressure. [1]

8. What fluids should we use? How much? What end points would I titrate to?

It is important to maintain high filling pressures; it doesn't matter what fluids initially.

You may need inotropic support if there is evidence of RV failure (as well as re-perfusion). [1]

Resuscitation should be titrated towards resolution of end organ or tissue hypoperfusion, guided by the ECG (ischaemia) urine output, base deficit or lactate. [1]

9. Which coronary territory has been affected?

It is usually the right coronary artery (RCA) but can be the circumflex artery from the left. [2]

10. What related clinical phenomena can occur with RCA infarcts?

There are varying degrees of atrioventricular conduction block. Around 40% of inferior myocardial infarctions are complicated by RV infarction. [2]

11. What are the indications for trans-venous pacing?

Indications for trans-venous pacing include refractory symptomatic bradycardia, Mobitz II secondary degree heart block (dropped beats), progressive type II or type III (complete) block associated with the ischaemia (*not* Wenckebach, this is Mobitz I and usually settles). [2]

12. What are the criteria for admission to an intensive care unit versus a coronary care unit?

Most coronary care units can manage inotropes and continuous positive airway pressure but the requirement for escalating or more complex cardiac, respiratory, renal or ventilatory support necessitates intensive care unit admission. [2]

13. This patient has had a PCI and a 'modern' coronary stent inserted. If the patient develops an acute abdomen 5 days later and needs a laparotomy, what are your concerns and what should you do about them?

You should carry out the usual pre-optimization and resuscitation. [1]

You need to know if they have a drug-eluting stent *in situ* and think about how to manage their antiplatelets and anticoagulation. You may need to suspend oral antiplatelet therapy and use intravenous antiplatelet bridging agents, which can be started and stopped much in the same way that intravenous heparin can. The risk of bleeding associated with residual antiplatelet effects may be outweighed by the risks of stent thrombosis. This requires close liaison with haematology, surgery, cardiology and anaesthesia. [1]

Data 37

A 23-year-old male is admitted to the intensive care unit post-operation following an uneventful but prolonged 10-hour neurosurgical procedure for a skull-based glomus tumour. He is otherwise fit and well with no other significant past medical history and normal baseline renal function. Eight hours later he is increasingly oliguric despite fluid challenges. He has remained haemodynamically stable throughout the perioperative period. There has been no response to bladder washout and renal ultrasound scan is reported as normal. His laboratory results are as follows:

		Reference range
Sodium	130 mmol/L	136–145 mmol/L
Potassium	6.5 mmol/L	3.6–5.2 mmol/L
Urea	13.4 mmol/L	2.5–6.4 mmol/L
Creatinine	158 µmol/L	80–132 µmol/L
Corrected calcium	1.95 mmol/L	2.10–2.65 mmol/L
Phosphate	2.4 mmol/L	0.7–1.4 mmol/L
WCC	15.2×10^9/L	$4–11 \times 10^9$/L
Haemoglobin	12.5 g/dL	11.5–16.5 g/dL
Platelets	143×10^9/L	$150–400 \times 10^9$/L
Albumin	30 g/L	35–50 g/L
Total bilirubin	14 umol/L	3–17 umol/L
AST	245 IU/L	15–37 IU/L
Alkaline phosphatase	90 IU/L	50–136 IU/L

1. **What do you think is the most likely cause for the above results and why?**
The results indicate rhabdomyolysis secondary to a compartment syndrome.   [3]
The history is suggestive of a possible compartment syndrome from the prolonged duration of surgery and likely immobilization. The classic biochemical picture of hyperkalaemia, hyperphosphatemia, hypocalcaemia and a high aspartate aminotransferase (AST) make rhabdomyolysis an important diagnosis to exclude.
Other differentials causing an acute kidney injury are unlikely.

2. What does his ECG demonstrate?

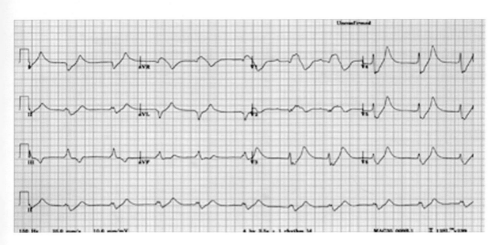

It shows tall T waves, broad QRS and absent P waves, suggestive of hyperkalaemia. [2]

3. What other tests would you like to do?
You could test the following:
- Urine for myoglobin [1]
- Creatinine kinase levels [1]
- Serum lactate dehydrogenase (LDH) [1]
- Arterial blood gas [1]
- Order a Doppler ultrasound scan of lower limbs [1]
- Measure the compartment pressures [1]

4. How would you treat rhabdomyolysis?
Treat the cause – for example fasciotomy if indicated. [1]

Ensure adequate hydration – you need generous amounts of fluid. [1]

Consider urinary alkalization with bicarbonate to keep pH > 6.5 (although there is limited evidence above fluid alone). [1]

Treat hyperkalaemia along conventional lines (ask for doses): [1]
- Calcium gluconate (typically 10 mL of 10%)
- Intravenous insulin/glucose (e.g. 10 units soluble insulin with 50 mL 50% glucose)
- Intravenous bicarbonate
- Nebulized salbutamol

Consider renal replacement therapy if indicated. [1]

5. What are the indications for acute renal replacement? [2 for all]
- Refractory hyperkalaemia
- Metabolic acidosis
- Volume overload with oligo/anuria
- Symptomatic uraemia (pericarditis, encephalopathy, bleeding)

6. What categories of drugs can cause this condition?   [1 for statins, 2 for all]

Examples include:

- Statins
- Serotonin syndrome caused by selective serotonin reuptake inhibitors (SSRIs)
- Drugs of abuse – cocaine, amphetamines, heroin, LSD, 'Ecstasy'

Data 38

This is the CT scan of a 55-year-old man who presents with sudden onset unilateral weakness and a low Glasgow Coma Scale (GCS).

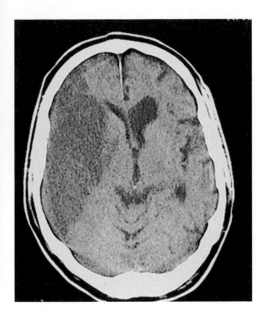

1. Describe the CT scan.

There is an extensive wedge-shaped area of low density in the right parietal lobe with some mass effect, indicated by compression of the right lateral ventricle and slight mid-line shift. This is likely to represent an acute middle cerebral artery infarct. [2]

2. How do you classify acute stroke?

Ischaemic strokes are either thrombotic or embolic and haemorrhagic strokes include intracerebral and subarachnoid haemorrhage. [1]

3. How would you initially assess a patient presenting with an acute stroke and low GCS? [3 for all]

You would carry out a standard airway, breathing and circulation assessment.

A disability assessment would include assessment of GCS, pupillary reaction, the presence of any focal neurological deficit including motor examination of tone, power, reflexes and plantar responses. You would assess for seizure activity.

You should check glucose levels.

Carry out a detailed history and examination, specifically looking for evidence of pro-thrombotic or haemorrhagic conditions, medications or cardiac sources of embolism and dysrhythmia.

4. Do you know of any scoring systems for patients with an acute stroke presenting to the emergency department? [2 for Rosier score and 1 for any other]

The ROSIER scoring system (Recognition Of Stroke In the Emergency Room) is a validated score. Positive scores (+1 for each) for new onset of:

- Asymmetric facial weakness
- Asymmetric arm weakness
- Asymmetric leg weakness
- Speech disturbance
- Visual field defect

Loss of consciousness/syncope or seizure activity score (–1) each. Stroke is likely if the total score is greater than 0.

Other scoring systems include the FAST (Face Arm Speech Test) or ABCD (age, blood pressure, clinical features, duration of transient ischaemic attack (TIA) and presence of diabetes) risk calculation tool following the TIA.

5. Is there a role for thrombolysis in acute stroke?

Yes! Early thrombolysis is recommended within 4.5 hours of an acute ischaemic stroke, provided intracranial haemorrhage has been excluded and no other contraindication to this exists. Not all centres can assess and thrombolyse acute stroke. [2]

6. What are the contraindications to thrombolysis? [2 for > 4, 3 for > 6]

Contraindications include:

- Seizure at onset of stroke
- Symptoms suggestive of subarachnoid haemorrhage
- Stroke or serious head injury in the preceding 3 months
- Major surgery or serious trauma within 2 weeks
- Previous intracranial haemorrhage
- Intracranial neoplasm
- Arteriovenous malformation or aneurysm
- Gastro-intestinal or urinary-tract haemorrhage in the preceding 3 weeks
- Current anticoagulation (INR > 1.7)

7. Are there any other medical therapies that we should initiate post stroke? [2 for all]

- Supportive care, which may include admission to the intensive care unit and assessment and control of ICP where appropriate
- Antiplatelet drug (as soon as haemorrhage has been excluded), e.g. aspirin
- Treatment of hyperglycaemia and fever, DVT prophylaxis (if no contraindications), attention to pressure areas and an early swallow assessment.

8. Should the patient's blood pressure be controlled acutely? [2 for all]

The current NICE stroke guidelines recommend anti-hypertensive treatment in people with acute stroke only if there is a hypertensive emergency with one or more of the following:

- Hypertensive encephalopathy
- Hypertensive nephropathy
- Hypertensive cardiac failure/myocardial infarction
- Aortic dissection
- Pre-eclampsia/eclampsia
- Intracerebral haemorrhage with systolic blood pressure over 200 mmHg

9. Is there a role for decompressive craniectomy?

There is limited evidence for the role of decompressive craniectomy as a control of raised intracranial pressure in the context of acute stroke but it could be considered alongside medical therapies such as cooling and thiopentone coma for patients with refractory intracranial hypertension. [2]

Data 39

You are asked to review a 48-year-old male on the haematology ward who has recently been diagnosed with acute myeloid leukaemia. His induction chemotherapy was commenced 2 days ago (continuous cytarabine infusion ongoing, and a daily dose of daunorubicin). He is also receiving allopurinol. Over the past few hours the patient has vomited three times and has complained of worsening muscle cramps. His urine output has been in the range of 5–10 mL per hour for the last 4 hours, during which he has received 3 litres of NaCl 0.9%. The latest observations are below:

Observation	Value
SpO$_2$ (FiO$_2$ 0.4)	96%
Respiratory rate	30/breaths/min
Heart rate	118 beats/min
Blood pressure	100/52 mmHg
Temperature	36.5 °C

His latest blood results are listed below.

		Reference range
Sodium	131 mmol/L	136–145 mmol/L
Potassium	7.9 mmol/L	3.6–5.2 mmol/L
Urea	14.2 mmol/L	2.5–6.4 mmol/L
Creatinine	353 µmol/L	80–132 µmol/L
WCC	14.4 × 10^9/L	4–11 × 10^9/L
Haemoglobin	8.4 g/dL	11.5–16.5 g/dL
Platelets	64 × 10^9/L	150–400 × 10^9/L
Uric acid	69.4 mg/dL	3.5–7.2 mg/dL
LDH	524 IU/L	140–280
Calcium^{++} (corrected)	1.7 mmol/L	2.25–2.5 mmol/L
Phosphate	3.6 mmol/L	0.8–1.4 mmol/L
FiO$_2$	0.21	
pH	7.14	7.35–7.45
pO$_2$	10.1 kPa	10.0–14 kPa

(cont.)

		Reference range
pCO$_2$	3.9 kPa	4.4–5.9 kPa
BE	−15.4 mEq/L	−2–(+2) mEq/L
Lactate	2.1 mmol/L	0–2 mmol/L

1. **Using the information you have been given, what do you think is the likely underlying problem? Can you list the key issues that need to addressed with this case?** [4 for all]

The underlying problem is likely to be tumour lysis syndrome (TLS). This is diagnosed on a laboratory basis with (two or more) high uric acid, potassium and phosphate, and low calcium following chemotherapy. Other features include a rising creatinine, cardiac arrhythmia or seizures.

The metabolic acidosis, thrombocytopenia and acute kidney injury are also concerns.

2. **What is TLS?** [2 for all]

TLS is an oncological emergency. It can be considered as a metabolic syndrome, characterized by rapid destruction of a large malignant cell load leading to release of significant amounts of intracellular components. The following facts are important:

- Hyperkalaemia can be life threatening
- Excess phosphate binds with calcium (leading to hypocalcaemia) leading to formation of calcium phosphate, which precipitates in tissues (including renal tubules)
- Nucleic acids break down to form uric acid

3. **What causes TLS?**

TLS occurs in malignancies associated with high tumour proliferation rate such as high-grade lymphomas and acute leukaemias with a significant tumour load. TLS may be spontaneous or secondary to chemotherapy, radiotherapy or more rarely glucocorticosteroid therapy. [2]

4. **What is the cause of acute kidney injury in TLS?**

Acute uric acid nephropathy involves deposition of uric acid crystals in the renal tubules, causing mechanical obstruction. Calcium phosphate is also deposited. [2]

5. **What are the principles of management you would use here?** [4 for all]

- ABCDE (airway, breathing, circulation, disability, exposure) initial approach
- Aggressive fluid therapy to maintain a high urine output (> 100 mL/kg per hour)
- Continuous cardiac monitoring
- Treatment of hyperkalaemia either medically or with renal replacement
  - Calcium gluconate
  - Insulin/dextrose
  - Nebulized salbutamol
  - Sodium bicarbonate
- Phosphate binder may be considered for hyperphosphataemia
- Rasburicase may have a role in hyperuricaemia refractory to resuscitation
- Hypocalcaemia
  - Calcium will be given as part of cardio-protective strategy for hyperkalaemia (as above)

- Hypocalcaemia correction has associated risk; in the presence of a high phosphate, correction of hypocalcaemia can encourage production of calcium phosphate, which can precipitate in the renal tubules and exacerbate the kidney injury
- Calcium replacement should be undertaken only if there are severe symptoms/complications (tetany, seizures, arrhythmias); aim is to treat complication, not normalize serum level
- Liaise closely with haematologist/oncologist

6. What is rasburicase? [2 for both]

Rasburicase is a recombinant form of urate oxidase. It catalyses the enzymatic oxidation of uric acid into allantoin (more soluble than uric acid), which is excreted by the kidneys. It is often used as prophylaxis if there is a high risk of TLS.

7. For what reasons could a patient with a haematological malignancy be referred to critical care? [2 for both]

A patient might be referred for management of complications related specifically to the malignancy or to its treatment (neutropenic sepsis, thrombocytopenia, hyperviscosity syndrome, chemotherapy induced mucositis, tumour lysis or organ toxicity).

They might also be referred to critical care for any unrelated coincidental medical or surgical condition.

8. Can you tell me about any specific complications directly related to specific chemotherapeutic agents? [1 for drug and complication to max. score 2]

The following chemotherapeutic agents can cause the complications indicated in parentheses:

- Bleomycin (pulmonary fibrosis)
- Cyclophosphamide (interstitial pneumonitis, haemorrhagic cystitis)
- Cytarabine (interstitial pneumonitis)
- Daunorubicin (cardiomyopathy)
- Vincristine (acute uric acid nephropathy, severe bronchospasm)

Data 40

These are the blood results from a 39-year-old man who has been admitted to intensive care with a community acquired pneumonia and septic shock. He has a past history of insulin-dependent diabetes mellitus and depression. He is currently ventilated and receiving vasopressors and renal replacement therapy. After 10 hours of aggressive haemofiltration he continues to have a refractory metabolic acidosis.

		Reference range
Sodium	144 mmol/L	136–145 mmol/L
Potassium	5.2 mmol/L	3.6–5.2 mmol/L
Urea	22.7 mmol/L	2.5–6.4 mmol/L
Creatinine	256 µmol/L	80–132 µmol/L
Albumin	21 g/L	35–50 g/L
Glucose	16 mmol/L	4.0–5.9 mmol/L
Total bilirubin	21 µmol/L	3–17 µmol/L
AST	66 IU/L	15–37 IU/L
Alkaline phosphatase	68 IU/L	50–136 IU/L
INR	1.3	
Haemoglobin	10.2 g/dL	11.5–16.5 g/dL
WCC	16.5×10^9/L	$4–11 \times 10^9$/L
Platelets	350×10^9/L	$150–400 \times 10^9$/L
FiO_2	0.65	
pH	7.25	7.35–7.45
pO_2	10.7 kPa	10.0–14 kPa
pCO_2	4.8 kPa	4.4–5.9 kPa
BE	−10.1 mEq/L	−2–(+2) mEq/L
Lactate	3.1 mmol/L	0–2 mmol/L
Bicarbonate	14 mmol/L	22–28 mmol/L

1. **What are the main differential diagnoses for the cause of his persistent acidosis and what further investigations would you request?**
- Hypoperfusion [1]
- Ongoing acute kidney injury [1]
- Diabetic ketoacidosis – check ketones [2]
- Hyperchloremic acidosis is a possibility (need chloride level) [2]
- Unmeasured anions – alcohol, methanol, ethylene glycol, salicylates [2]

2. **His serum chloride levels are 110 mmol/L – calculate the anion gap.**

$$\text{Anion gap} = (Na^+ + K^+) - (Cl^- + HCO_3^-) = (144 + 5.2) - (110 + 14) = 25.2$$

Normal ranges depend on measurement but are widely considered as 8 to 16 mEq/L plasma when not including $[K^+]$ and from 10 to 20 mEq/L otherwise. This patient has a raised anion gap metabolic acidosis. [2]

3. **His serum ketones levels are 7.5 mg/dL (normal is < 1 mg/dL). How would you manage this?**

Start a fixed-rate intravenous insulin infusion (FRIII) calculated on 0.1 units per kilogram body weight to normalize glucose levels and aid clearance of ketones. [1]

Carry out fluid replacement with normal saline or balanced crystalloid to restore circulatory volume. [1]

Use an intravenous infusion of 10% glucose in order to avoid hypoglycaemia and permit the continuation of an FRIII to suppress ketogenesis. This is recommended when the blood glucose falls below 14.0 mmol/L and given along with standard fluid resuscitation. [1]

Correct any electrolyte imbalance. Serum potassium is often high initially (although total body potassium is low) and can fall rapidly after commencing treatment with insulin. Regular monitoring is essential. Monitor and correct hypophosphataemia. [1]

4. **What treatment targets would you aim for?** [1 for some, 2 for all]

The recommended targets (from the Joint British Diabetes Society guidelines for the management of diabetic ketoacidosis) are:
- Blood glucose reducing by 3.0 mmol/L per hour
- A fall in blood ketone concentration by 0.5 mmol/L per hour
- Increasing venous bicarbonate by 3.0 mmol/L per hour
- Maintain potassium between 4.0 and 5.5 mmol/L

5. **What would you do if your targets were not being met?**

If these rates are not achieved, then the FRIII rate should be increased. [1]

6. **Would you use a bicarbonate infusion? Why/Why not?** [1 for 'no' and 1 for explanation]

Adequate fluid and insulin therapy will resolve the acidosis in diabetic ketoacidosis (DKA) and the use of bicarbonate is not indicated (in current guidelines). The acidosis may be an adaptive response as it improves oxygen delivery to the tissues by causing a right shift of the oxygen dissociation curve. Excessive bicarbonate may cause a rise in the CO_2 partial pressure in the cerebrospinal fluid (CSF) and may lead to a paradoxical increase in CSF acidosis. In addition, the use of bicarbonate in DKA may delay the fall in blood lactate: pyruvate ratio and ketones when compared to intravenous 0.9% sodium chloride. There are reports of bicarbonate contributing to cerebral oedema in children and young adults.

7. **What upper limit blood sugar target do you normally aim for in general for your critical care patients?**

The recommended upper glucose target is 10 mmol/L. Both hyper- and hypoglycaemia are associated with increased morbidity and mortality. The NICE–SUGAR study (*NEJM* 2009; 360: 1283–1297) compared intensive versus conventional glycemic control and found an excess mortality and higher frequency of hypoglycaemic episodes in the former group. [1]

Data 41

A 70-year-old lady has been transferred to your unit from the cardiac intensive care unit. She is now day 8 post coronary artery bypass grafting (CABG) and is struggling to wean from mechanical ventilation. She has a background history of heart failure and mild chronic obstructive pulmonary disease (COPD).

1. This is her ECG taken during a spontaneous breathing trial. What does it show?

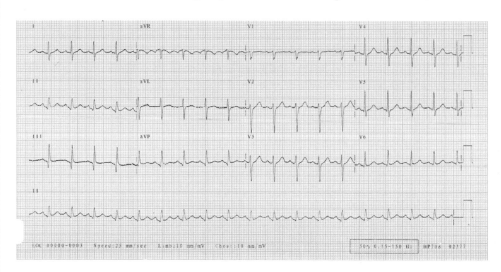

It shows sinus tachycardia with a rate of approximately 120 beats per minute. The axis is normal. QRS morphology is normal with minimal ST elevation in the inferior leads. This could represent early ischaemia during the stress of the spontaneous breathing trial.   [2]

2. **How do you define a 'failure to wean'?**
Prolonged weaning can be defined as failing three or more spontaneous breathing trials (SBTs) or requiring more than 7 days of mechanical ventilation following the first SBT.   [2]

3. **What initial investigations would you consider to help with your management?**
[up to 4 marks]

Search for and treat infection: check the full blood count (FBC) and C-reactive protein (CRP), send blood and respiratory tract cultures.

Exclude metabolic causes for weakness: review urea and electrolytes (U&E), liver function test (LFT), phosphate and magnesium levels.

Assess cardiac function: echocardiography and B-type natriuretic peptide (BNP) levels can give an indication of heart failure.

Assess coexisting respiratory pathology: chest X-ray and/or chest CT scan.

Exclude neuromuscular conditions, e.g. by electromyography (EMG), check for autoantibodies.

4. Can you describe general principles you would use to maximize chances of a successful wean? [up to 4 marks]

Aim to optimize cardiac and respiratory status – for example treat associated factors such as heart failure, fluid overload and infection.

Optimize nutritional status, glucose control and correct electrolyte imbalance.

Exclude underlying neuromuscular disorders.

Create weaning plans/diaries.

Set up sedation protocols.

Be consistent in approach with regard to the method of wean, avoid weaning at night.

Extubation onto non-invasive ventilation (NIV) may be considered in appropriate cases.

Facilitate early mobilization and rehabilitation.

5. This patient has had a transthoracic echocardiogram, which has revealed the presence of a normal ejection fraction, evidence of left ventricular hypertrophy, a dilated left atrium and abnormal mitral inflow and tissue Doppler studies. What diagnosis could be a contributory cause for her failure to wean?

The above findings strongly suggest the presence of diastolic dysfunction as a potential cause. [2]

6. What is critical illness neuromyopathy?

Critical illness neuromyopathy (CINM) is a term used to describe the association of muscle weakness and polyneuropathy associated with critical illness. It is a common cause of intensive care unit acquired weakness. [1]

7. What clinical features would suggest this diagnosis?

Diagnosis is initially based on clinical features including weakness and wasting, usually symmetric weakness, hyporeflexia and hypotonia. Associated sensory signs may be difficult to elicit. Cranial nerve signs are usually not a feature. [2]

8. How would you confirm your diagnosis? [3 for all, 2 for most]

The diagnosis is largely clinical but confirmatory tests may be necessary.

Nerve conduction studies show a reduction in amplitude of compound muscle and/or sensory nerve action potentials with preserved conduction velocity.

EMG may show either low or normal compound muscle action potentials.

Carry out a muscle biopsy to aid the diagnosis of myopathy (abnormal, atrophic myofibres with filament loss +/– necrosis) and exclude other causes.

Consider MRI to exclude other pathology such as cord and brainstem lesions.

Creatine kinase levels may be normal or raised.

Data 42

This is the chest X-ray of a 55-year-old man who has presented with a 3-week history of increasing shortness of breath. He has been recently under review with his GP and has had two courses of antibiotics with no benefit. He has been admitted to hospital and treated for a severe community-acquired pneumonia.

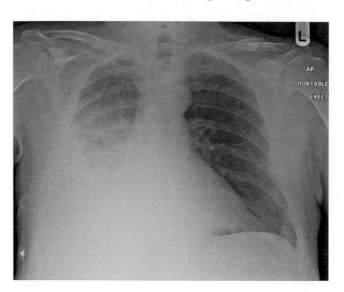

1. Comment on the chest X-ray.

It shows the anteroposterior (AP) erect chest film, adequately exposed and orientated. There is a large right-sided pleural effusion occupying two thirds of the lung field.   [1]

2. What additional investigations would you arrange for?

Carry out the following blood tests: full blood count (FBC), urea and electrolytes (U&Es), liver function tests (LFTs), lactate dehydrogenase (LDH), glucose, clotting and C-reactive protein (CRP).   [1]

Order/perform an ultrasound scan, which improves the success rate of aspiration and aids the detection of septations.   [1]

Carry out a pleural fluid aspiration procedure.   [1]

A CT scan at some point will help to identify the size extent of any loculations or pleural thickening. Consider bronchoscopy if there is a concern of underlying malignancy and for broncho-alveolar lavage.   [1 for either/both]

3. What causes pleural effusions?   [2 for all]

Transudates or exudates can cause pleural effusions.

Transudates are more common and occur when the balance between oncotic pressures and hydrostatic pressure is disrupted, leading to interstitial fluid accumulating in the pleural space. Common causes include congestive heart failure, liver cirrhosis, nephrotic syndrome, myxoedema or any hypoproteinaemic state.

Exudates are usually due to infection, trauma or inflammation. Examples include pulmonary infection, trauma, pulmonary infarction, pulmonary embolism, autoimmune disorders, pancreatitis, ruptured oesophagus (Boerhaave's syndrome), tuberculosis or following thoracic surgery. Lung cancer, breast cancer, and lymphoma cause around 75% of all malignant pleural effusions.

4. Talk me through how you would do a pleural tap. [2 for all]

Obtain consent if you are able to, otherwise consider consent 'Form 4'. (Always get consent in an examination!)

Confirm the correct side and review radiology.

Make sure the procedure is ultrasound-guided.

Administer local anaesthesia.

Ensure full asepsis.

Patients should be appropriately monitored and trained assistance should be available.

The preferred site for needle insertion is the triangle of safety (see question 5) with the needle inserted just above the rib to avoid the neurovascular bundle.

5. What tests would you do on pleural fluid? [3 for all, 2 for most]

You would carry out microscopy, culture and sensitivity tests including urgent Gram stain and testing for acid-fast bacilli (e.g. tuberculosis).

Amylase is elevated in oesophageal rupture, pancreatitis or cancer.

Glucose is decreased with cancer, bacterial infections or rheumatoid pleuritis.

Pleural fluid pH is low in empyema (< 7.2) and may be low in some cancers (you can process through a blood gas analyser for a quick result).

Cytology is indicated if there is suspicion of malignancy.

Pleural fluid albumin and LDH can help determine exudative or transudative causes.

6. What are Light's criteria?

These help to determine the aetiology. The criteria below are consistent with an exudate:

- Pleural fluid serum protein ratio more than 0.5 [1]
- Pleural fluid serum LDH ratio more than 0.6 [1]
- Pleural fluid LDH more than two thirds of normal serum value [1]

7. Here are the results – please can you comment on them.

Serum protein = 50g/L   Pleural fluid protein = 30 g/L

Serum LDH = 180 IU/L   Pleural fluid LDH = 140 IU/L

Pleural pH = 7.1

The above results are consistent with an exudate. [1]

8. How would you manage this?

Investigate and treat the cause – in this case it is likely secondary to pneumonia. [1]

Consider drainage of effusion. [1]

9. You have inserted a 'Seldinger' chest drain, with only minimal drainage of pleural fluid. What steps will you take? [2 for all, 1 for 2]

Consider whether the effusion is simple or complex. This may require further imaging and help from respiratory or cardiothoracic colleagues. Options include:

- Wide-bore chest drain
- CT guided drainage – if it doesn't drain you need to see where tube is positioned
- Video-assisted placement (video-assisted thoracic surgery (VATS) procedure)
- Consider intra-pleural fibrinolytics such as tissue plasminogen activator (tPA) or DNA-ase

Data 43

A 52-year-old man is being reviewed at the intensive care unit follow-up clinic. He has a past history of alcohol excess and stage 3 chronic kidney disease. He was discharged 6 weeks ago after a week's stay in critical care with severe sepsis and acute kidney injury (AKI) secondary to a pneumonia. His main complaint currently is that of shortness of breath and fatigue. These are blood results performed recently by his GP.

		Reference range
WCC	4.5×10^9/L	4–11×10^9/L
Haemoglobin	8.9 g/dL	11.5–16.5 g/dL
Platelets	125×10^9/L	150–400×10^9/L

1. What are the main abnormalities?
The blood results show a low haemoglobin (Hb) concentration and borderline low platelet count. [1]

2. What information regarding the Hb concentration is missing from the full blood count? [1 for all]
Standard information including the mean corpuscular volume (MCV), mean corpuscular haemoglobin (MCH) and mean corpuscular haemoglobin concentration (MCHC) are missing.

3. How do you define anaemia? [1 for both]
The commonly used definition from the World Health Organization is the following:
- Men Hb < 130g/L
- Women Hb < 120g/L

4. How can the MCV help us?
The MCV is used to classify anaemias into microcytic (< 80 fL), normocytic (80–95 fL) and macrocytic (95–105 fL) (note fL = 10^{-15} L). [1]

5. Can you name some likely possible causes for his anaemia. [1 for structure, up to 3 for answers]
There are multiple possible causes for his anaemia, broadly classified into red-cell production problems, bleeding (loss of cells) and reduced lifespan in the circulation due to destruction of red cells.
- Anaemia related to haemopoietic deficiency – iron deficiency may be contributed to by poor dietary intake, malabsorption or occult blood loss and causes a microcytic hypochromic anaemia
- B12/folate deficiency related to poor dietary intake, malabsorption and alcoholism results in a macrocytic anaemia
- Anaemia of chronic disease – he has a past history of alcohol excess and chronic kidney disease. Alcohol excess is associated with direct toxic effects on the bone marrow and chronic liver disease. This is often a normochromic normocytic anaemia

- Gastro-intestinal (GI) blood loss
- Anaemia resulting from his recent critical illness and contributed to by interventions performed during his recent admission (haemodilution, blood sampling/haemofiltration)
- Haemolysis is a less likely cause

6. How would you investigate this in the follow-up clinic? [4 for all]

Carry out iron studies – including ferritin, transferrin, total iron binding capacity (TIBC) and transferrin saturation.

A low ferritin level accompanied by raised transferrin and TIBC levels, with low transferrin saturation is a feature of iron deficiency.

Check B12/folate levels.

Do urea and electrolytes (U&Es) and liver function tests (LFTs).

Carry out a faecal occult blood test if you suspect GI blood loss.

7. What are the problems in investigating anaemia in critical care patients?

The acute inflammatory process interferes with the interpretation of tests; for example, ferritin is an acute stage protein and levels are often raised secondary to inflammation whereas transferrin levels and the TIBC are often reduced. [2]

8. How does haemoglobin influence oxygen delivery?

This is an equation you must know!

$$\text{Oxygen delivery} = CO \times CaO_2;$$

$$CaO_2 = (Hb \times SaO_2 \times 1.39) + (0.003 \times PaO_2)$$

where CO = cardiac output, CaO_2 = arterial oxygen content, SaO_2 = oxygen saturation and PaO_2 is the partial pressure of oxygen in the arterial blood. [2]

9. What transfusion thresholds would you apply to a patient in critical care and what is the evidence for this approach? [3 for all]

Current guidelines are in favour of restrictive transfusion practices aimed at keeping Hb levels > 70 g/L. The evidence for this comes largely from the results of two randomized controlled trials – the TRICC (*NEJM* 1999; 340: 409–417) and TRISS (*NEJM* 2014; 371: 1381–391) trials.

The TRICC trial compared a restrictive strategy (Hb < 7 g/dL) versus a liberal transfusion strategy (Hb < 10 g/dL). Overall 30-day mortality was similar in both groups; however, a significant survival benefit was seen in patients in the restrictive strategy cohort who were less acutely ill and those below 55 years of age.

The TRISS trial recruited patients with septic shock; compared restrictive (Hb < 7 g/dL) and liberal(Hb < 9 g/dL) strategies showed no difference in the primary outcome of 90-day mortality between groups.

10. What exclusions would you apply to the above principle?

Patients with ongoing active bleeding are an exception to this rule. Patients with active coronary ischaemia should also be managed on a case-by-case basis. [1]

Data 44

60-year-old male presents to hospital with malaise, nausea and jaundice but no clear precipitant. Past medical history is insignificant apart from a history of depression. He is increasingly confused. General examination is unremarkable apart from the presence of a mild tachycardia and jaundice. Routine blood tests at his GP, 3 weeks ago, were normal.

		Reference range
Sodium	133 mmol/L	136–145 mmol/L
Potassium	5.7 mmol/L	3.6–5.2 mmol/L
Chloride	105 mmol/L	100–108 mmol/L
Urea	14.7 mmol/L	2.5–6.4 mmol/L
Creatinine	161 µmol/L	80–132µmol/L
Total protein	79 g/L	64–82 g/L
Albumin	38 g/L	35–50 g/L
Globulin	41g/L	23–35 g/L
Total bilirubin	89 µmol/L	3–17 µmol/L
Conjugated bilirubin	52 µmol/L	0–3 µmol/L
ALT	224 IU/L	30–65 IU/L
AST	359 IU/L	15–37 IU/L
Alkaline phosphatase	83 IU/L	50–136 IU/L
Gamma glutamyl transferase (GT)	31 IU/L	15–85 IU/L

1. What do you think could be the problem?
The blood results show evidence of deranged liver function, acute kidney injury and hyperkalaemia. These are acute abnormalities given his recent blood tests were reported as normal. [1]

2. How do you define acute liver failure? Can you classify it.
Jaundice, encephalopathy and coagulopathy are the three main features. [1]
It can be classified into hyperacute, acute and subacute: [1]
    Hyperacute – less than 7 days from jaundice to encephalopathy

Acute – jaundice to encephalopathy time is less than 28 days
Subacute – jaundice to encephalopathy time is less than 6 months.

3. **Give a differential diagnosis for the causes of acute liver failure.** [1 each for first 2, 2 for the rest]

- Drug-induced liver disease – paracetamol being the commonest in the UK
- Viral hepatitis – Hepatitis A, B, C and E
- Alcoholic hepatitis [2 for most]
- Autoimmune hepatitis
- Miscellaneous – ischaemic hepatitis, Budd Chiari (hepatic venous obstruction: classical triad of abdominal pain, ascites and liver enlargement), malignancy, HELLP syndrome (haemolysis, elevated liver enzymes and low platelets in late pregnancy), acute fatty liver of pregnancy, Wilson's disease (autosomal recessive disorder of copper transportation)

4. **What other laboratory results would you request?** [max. 5]

- Clotting studies
- Arterial blood gas including lactate/glucose levels
- Paracetamol/salicylate levels
- Autoimmune screen – anti smooth muscle and anti mitochondrial antibodies
- Viral hepatitis screen
- Serum ammonia levels

Further information is now offered to candidates. The following results are subsequently received:

		Reference range		
INR	3.2	< 1.3	pH	7.25
APTT ratio	2.1		pO_2	11 kPa
Fibrinogen	70 mg/dL	200–400 mg/dL	pCO_2	4.3 kPa
Lactate	4.1 mmol/L	0–2 mmol/L	Bicarbonate	16 mmol/L
Glucose	2.6 mmol/L	4.4–6.1 mmol/L	BXS	−8.1
Ammonia	85	15–45 µg/dL		
Salicylates	undetected			
Paracetamol	21 mg/L	See normogram		

5. **What immediate actions would you take?**
Start N-acetylcysteine (NAC) as paracetamol levels are elevated, there is uncertainty around the time of ingestion and, with the deranged liver function tests (LFTs), this is likely to be a delayed presentation. [1]
Correct the hypoglycaemia, with bolus and infusion of intravenous dextrose. [1]

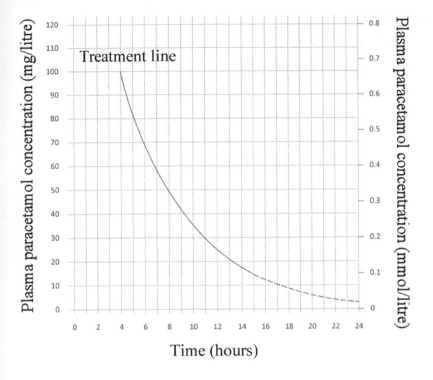

6. **He deteriorates over the next 24 hours and becomes increasingly confused. How do we grade hepatic encephalopathy?**

The West Haven Grading system is most commonly used: [2]

- Grade 0: subclinical; normal mental status, but minimal changes in memory, concentration, intellectual function, co-ordination; this is also termed minimal hepatic encephalopathy
- Grade 1: mild confusion, euphoria or depression, decreased attention, slowing of ability to perform mental tasks, irritability, disorder of sleep pattern such as inverted sleep cycle
- Grade 2: drowsiness, lethargy, gross deficits in ability to perform mental tasks, obvious personality changes, inappropriate behaviour, intermittent disorientation
- Grade 3: somnolent but rousable, unable to perform mental tasks, disorientation to time and place, marked confusion, amnesia, occasional fits of rage, speech present but incomprehensible
- Grade 4: coma, with or without response to painful stimuli; decorticate or decerebrate posturing

7. **A CT scan of the brain is ordered. What does it show?**

The scan shows widespread loss of grey–white matter differentiation consistent with cerebral oedema. [1]

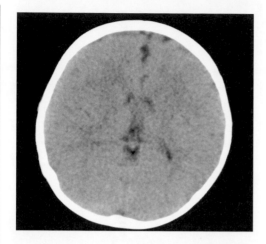

8. What are the priorities in managing the cerebral oedema? [3 for all]

- Head-up tilt
- Normocapnia
- Maintain cerebral perfusion pressure (MAP – ICP, i.e. the difference between the mean arterial pressure and the intracranial pressure)
- Consider ICP monitor to guide targeted therapy
- Normoglycaemia
- Transfer to a specialist centre

Data 45

A 45-year-old female is admitted to the emergency department at 21:30, with a history of four episodes of 'coffee ground vomiting' over the last 24 hours. Her husband called an ambulance following an episode of vomiting in which a large amount of fresh blood was evident. The notes available reveal alcohol excess (known liver cirrhosis), previous intravenous recreational drug use, anxiety and depression. On arrival she is noted to have a Glasgow Coma Scale (GCS) score of 13 (M6 V4 E3). The following observations are recorded:

Observation	Value
SpO$_2$ (FiO$_2$ 0.35)	97%
Respiratory rate	24 breaths/min
Heart rate	115 beats/min
Blood pressure	95/43 mmHg

Her initial blood results are listed below.

		Reference range
Sodium	129 mmol/L	136–145 mmol/L
Potassium	3.4 mmol/L	3.6–5.2 mmol/L
Urea	24.2 mmol/L	2.5–6.4 mmol/L
Creatinine	121 µmol/L	80–132 µmol/L
WCC	14.3 × 10^9/L	4–11 × 10^9/L
Haemoglobin	7.8 g/dL	11.5–16.5 g/dL
Platelets	63 × 10^9/L	150–400 × 10^9/L
Albumin	24 g/L	35–50 g/L
Total bilirubin	61 µmol/L	3–17 µmol/L
ALT	78 IU/L	30–65 IU/L
AST	67 IU/L	15–37 IU/L
INR	2.8	
APTT	35 seconds	28–38 seconds
FiO$_2$	0.21	
pH	7.28	7.35–7.45
pO$_2$	9.7 kPa	10.0–14 kPa
pCO$_2$	5.6 kPa	4.4–5.9 kPa
BE	−6.9 mEq/L	−2–(+2) mEq/L
Bicarbonate	18 mmol/L	22–28 mmol/L
Lactate	4.7 mmol/L	0–2 mmol/L

1. **What are the major issues in this case?** [2 for most]
- Upper gastro-intestinal (GI) bleed (known liver cirrhosis – likely variceal bleed)
- Haemodynamics – mild hypotension, tachycardia
- Anaemia
- Coagulopathy
  - Thrombocytopenia
  - Raised INR
- Altered conscious level (possible hepatic encephalopathy)
- Abnormal hepatic blood results
  - Raised INR
  - Low albumin
  - Raised bilirubin/ALT/AST
  - Lactic acidosis
- Previous intravenous drug use
  - Risk of blood-borne infection – a need for personal protective equipment
  - Difficult intravenous access

2. **What are the causes of upper GI bleeding?** [2 for all, 1 for most]
- Peptic ulcer (gastric or duodenal)
- Oesophagitis/gastritis/duodenitis
- Oesophageal/gastric varices
- Mallory–Weiss syndrome
- Angiodysplasia
- Aorto-enteric fistula
- Malignancy (oesophageal/gastric)

3. **What further information regarding this case would you like?** [3 for all, 2 for most]
- Confirm history of events and PMH
  - Medications (non-steroidal anti-inflammatory drugs, corticosteroids, antiplatelets, anticoagulants)
  - Alcohol history
  - Previous GI bleeds
  - History of liver disease (e.g. previous variceal bleeds)
  - Viral status (hepatitis)
- Examination
  - Evidence of chronic liver disease
  - Abdominal examination – assess for possible surgical cause
- Investigations
  - Previous liver function tests
  - Previous liver imaging (CT/ultrasound)
  - Previous endoscopy findings

4. **How would you manage the clotting abnormalities in this case?** [1 for most]
There is always a balance, especially if the patient may be a liver transplant candidate (and needs to meet biochemical transplant criteria). However, in an *actively bleeding* patient:

Transfuse fresh frozen plasma if INR > 1.5.

Transfuse platelets if platelet count $< 50 \times 10^9$/L.

If a massive haemorrhage is suspected, transfuse as per massive haemorrhage protocols.

5. **What pharmacological therapies would you consider in this case?** [3 for all, 2 for most]
- Terlipressin
- Proton pump inhibitor, e.g. high-dose omeprazole, or infusion
- Tranexamic acid
- Broad spectrum antibiotic, e.g. ceftriaxone
- Prokinetics, e.g. erythromycin – promotes gastric emptying, thus reducing the need for second look endoscopy.
- Thiamine to reduce potential for encephalopathy
- Lactulose (may reduce risk of hepatic encephalopathy – consider nasogastric administration balancing risks and benefits of nasogastric tube insertion)

6. **What is terlipresin and how does it work?** [2 for all, 1 for most]

Terlipressin (Triglycyl-lysine-vasopressin) is a pro-drug of vasopressin.

It acts on V1 receptors.

It causes splanchnic vasoconstriction leading to reduced portal blood flow and portal pressure, which in turn leads to reduced variceal pressure.

It has some side effects, including increased systemic vascular resistance, reduced cardiac output and reduced coronary blood flow.

7. **The patient has a further large episode of haematemesis. She loses consciousness and becomes haemodynamically unstable (blood pressure 70/40 mmHg, heart rate 135 beats per minute). How would you manage the situation?** [2 for all, 1 for most]
- Call for help (intensive care unit consultant, anaesthetist, gastroenterologist on call for endoscopy)
- Activate massive haemorrhage protocol
- Check airway, breathing, circulation
- Utilize principles of permissive hypotension
- Secure the airway with an endotracheal tube
  - Personal protective equipment (face-mask with visor)
  - Rapid sequence induction
    - Pre-oxygenate
    - Cricoid pressure
    - Full monitoring (SpO$_2$, ECG, non-invasive blood pressure, CO$_2$)
  - Anticipate possible difficulty with blood in the oropharynx
  - Induction agent choice – justified in presence of haemodynamic instability
- Consider transfer to theatre
- Need for urgent upper GI endoscopy (not often immediately available)
- Sengstaken–Blakemore tube as temporizing measure

8. **Can you identify the key features of a Sengstaken–Blakemore (SB) tube and describe how you would safely use it in an intubated patient?**

Note: The Sengstaken tube has ports for oesophageal and gastric balloons and a gastric aspiration port. The Minnesota tube has, in addition, an oesophageal aspiration port. [1]

Use a stepwise approach to safe insertion. [2]

Pre-insertion
1. Test inflate gastric and oesophageal balloons, using 50 a mL syringe filled with air. Following the test ensure both balloons are fully deflated.
2. Lubricate the tube.

Insertion
1. It can be inserted blindly (similar to a nasogastric tube); however the use of a laryngo-scope is preferable.
2. Advance the tube in until the 50 cm mark at the level of the teeth.

Position check
1. Inject 20 mL of air into the gastric aspiration lumen and listen with a stethoscope over the stomach.
2. Inflate the gastric balloon with 50 mL of air.
3. Get a chest X-ray to confirm the correct position (gastric balloon below the diaphragm, in the stomach).

Full SB tube deployment
1. Once the correct SB tube position is confirmed on the chest X-ray, fully inflate the gastric balloon (a total 250 mL of air) using 50-mL syringes.
2. Apply traction to the SB tube using a 500 mL bag of intravenous fluid.
3. Make a note of the depth at the teeth (this allows monitoring for SB tube displacement).

Assessment of bleeding
1. Apply suction to the gastric aspiration lumen and empty the stomach of blood.
2. Lavage the stomach – inject 50 mL NaCl 0.9% and aspirate. This can be repeated. You can attempt to assess if active bleeding is occurring below the gastric balloon.
3. Apply suction to the oesophageal aspiration lumen; if no blood is aspirated, you can stop here. If there is evidence of bleeding in the oesophagus, inflate the oesophageal balloon with air to a pressure of 40 mmHg, using a sphygmomanometer.
4. The oesophageal balloon should be deflated for 5 minutes every hour.

9. What are the complications associated with using an SB tube?
A possible complication is aspiration. This can be avoided if the patient is intubated.   [1]
There is also a risk of oesophageal injury: from *perforation* if you fully inflate the gastric balloon in the oesophagus; or from *mucosal ischaemia* if there is excessive oesophageal balloon pressure or if it is inflated for a long duration.   [1]

Data 46

A 30-year-old man is admitted to critical care with a severe head injury and cerebral contusions. He has been sedated, intubated and ventilated for 4 days. Have a look at this part of the intensive care chart.

1. What has happened during the period shown?

Infusions (Drug Dosage Rate, i.e. mgs/hr, mmols/hr, iu/hr)										
PROPOFOL	mg/hr	200	180	150	OFF	OFF	OFF	300	180	
ALFENTANIL	mg/hr	2	2	1	OFF	OFF	OFF	3	2	

	MODE	SIMV	SIMV	SIMV	CPAP/PS	CPAP/PS	CPAP/PS	SIMV	SIMV	
	FiO2	.5	.5	.4	.4	.5	.8	.7	.7	
	P peak/PEEP	25 6	25 6	25 6	20 5	15 5	12 5	26 6	28 6	
	MV/TV	450	480	460	420	660	380	690	470	
	f set/meas	16 16	16 16	16 16	8	12	33	16 16	16 16	
(Red)	SpO2	96	95	96	95	95	92	97	98	
(Cuff Pressure) in green	Air Entry									
	Sputum	/	/	min	/	/	min	/	/	
	Suction			✓			✓			
	Sedation Score	-3	-2	-2	-1	0	+3	-4	-3	

INPUT										
Crystalloid	Hartmans.	125	125	125	125	125	125	125	125	
NG feed										
IV/NG Drugs										
Co-Amoxyclav			250ml.							
PROPOFOL		20	18	15	/	/	/	30	18	
ALFENTANIL		2	2	1	/	/	/	3	2	

The propofol and alfentanil sedation has been temporarily stopped with a resulting rise in conscious level. The patient then becomes agitated and is re-sedated.   [2]

2. Why do we use sedation in intensive care?
Sedatives are used to improve patient comfort, decrease anxiety, permit mechanical ventilation and help facilitate interventions.   [1]

3. Why do we do sedation holds?   [4 for all]
Sedation agents cause haemodynamic compromise and can prolong recovery. It is fairly easy to completely over-sedate a patient such that when you decide to stop sedation it may take several days to wear off. There are no rapidly available tests to measure plasma levels of common sedative agents. Other effects of prolonged sedation include:

- Prolonged mechanical ventilation
- Gastric stasis
- Immune suppression
- Organ toxicity
- Difficulty in assessing neurological status
- Increased risk of ventilator acquired pneumonia
- Increased risk of venous thrombo-embolism
- Upper gastro-intestinal bleeding

4. Other than sedation holds, how else can we titrate sedation?
Excessive sedation can be avoided by titrating sedation to the optimal level of patient comfort. This is achieved using bedside sedation scoring systems. Some units use depth of anaesthesia monitoring, which are usually modified electroencephalogram (EEG) analysis, bispectral index (BIS) monitors or E-entropy. [2]

4. Can you give me an example of a sedation scoring system and how it is used? [2]
The Richmond Agitation Sedation Score (RASS) is a commonly used scoring system, detailed below. Other common examples include the Ramsay Sedation Scale and the Riker Sedation Agitation Scale (SAS).

   RASS:
- +4 Combative
- +3 Very agitated
- +2 Agitated
- +1 Restless
- 0 Alert and calm
- −1 Drowsy
- −2 Light sedation
- −3 Moderate sedation
- −4 Deep sedation to physical stimulation
- −5 Unarousable

5. Are there any situations in which you would not wish to perform a sedation hold?
[score 1 for each to maximum of 4]
- Raised intracranial pressure (ICP) (without direct ICP monitoring)
- Neuromuscular blockade
- Certain modes of mechanical ventilation that are unpleasant to tolerate (reverse ratio, airway pressure release ventilation)
- If the patient has a critical airway device or procedure that requires minimal movement (e.g. complex skin grafting).
- Prone positioning
- Severe hypoxia or high airway pressures

6. Are there any proven benefits of sedation holds in the intensive care unit literature?
Sedation holds with spontaneous breathing trials have been shown to significantly reduce duration on mechanical ventilation and the intensive care unit length of stay. (The Girard and Kress trial is probably the best known (*Lancet* 2008; 371: 126–134.) [2]

6. Calculate the 'safe' dose of propofol for a 70-kg adult.
The recommended maximum safe dose is 4 mg/kg per hour. Higher doses risk the complications of over-sedation, and also propofol-infusion syndrome. Cases have

been reported with lower doses than this. In a 70-kg adult this works out to 280 mg per hour which is equivalent to 28 mL of 1% propofol per hour. [2]

7. How does propofol contribute to calorie intake?

Propofol contains 1.1 kcal/mL and can significantly contribute to calorie intake and this needs to be taken into account when working out daily calorie requirements. [1]

Data 47

This is the electroencephalogram (EEG) of a 54-year-old man who has been admitted to critical care with increasing drowsiness, confusion and altered behaviour. He has a background of alcohol excess. A CT brain scan performed on admission was reported as normal.

1. What does the EEG show?

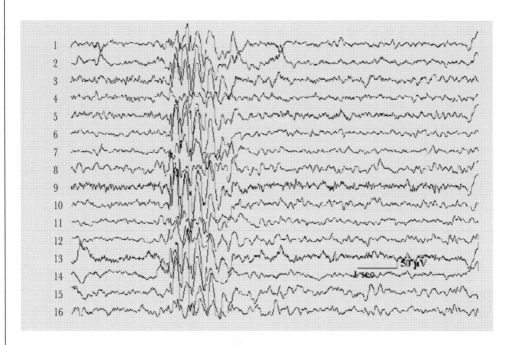

The EEG shows characteristic 'spike and wave' seizure activity. This is focal and not generalized. [2]

2. What waveforms are seen on the normal EEG? [1 for all, 2 for detail]
- Delta: 1–3Hz (non-rapid-eye-movement (REM) sleep)
- Theta: 4–7Hz (REM sleep)
- Alpha: 8–15Hz (awake with closed eyes, relaxing)
- Beta: 15–30Hz (full alertness)

3. What additional tests would you like to have available to help make a diagnosis?
Full blood count, urea and electroytes (U&Es), liver function test, glucose [1]
- Toxicology screen [1]
- Consider repeating CT brain scan [1]
- Lumbar puncture if no contraindications [1]

4. **The microbiology lab telephones the results of the cerebrospinal fluid (CSF) below. What is the most likely diagnosis?**

	CSF sample	Normal range
Colour	Clear	Clear
White cells (per mm³)	125	< 5
Differential	Lymphocytes	
CSF plasma:glucose ratio	71%	66% (approx)
Protein g/L	0.71	< 0.45

The most likely diagnosis is viral encephalitis. [1]

5. **What contraindications are there to lumbar puncture?**
The presence of a coagulopathy; most would consider a platelet count of $< 50 \times 10^9/L$ or INR > 1.5 as risk factors for bleeding. Medication with aspirin is considered relatively safe to perform a lumbar puncture whereas other antiplatelet agents (such as clopidogrel or ticlodipine) are usually considered unsafe. Confirmed or suspected raised intracranial pressure and local infection are also common contraindications. [2]

6. **What are alternative diagnostic tests in this situation?**   [2 for both]
Blood polymerase chain reaction (PCR) and antibody testing is possible, but this is less useful in the acute phase.
An MRI brain scan is another alternative diagnostic tool.

7. **What does the MRI scan below show?**

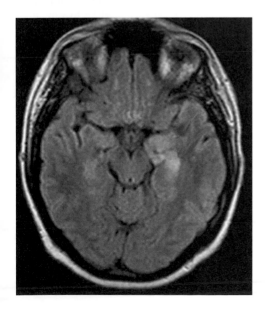

MRI appearances are characteristic and here the appearance manifests as bilateral asymmetrical involvement of the limbic system, medial temporal lobes and inferolateral frontal lobes. This image shows MRI fluid-attenuated inversion recovery (FLAIR) and demonstrates a bilateral medial temporal lobe hyperintense signal, predominantly involving the left hippocampus. [2]

8. What organisms could cause viral encephalitis? [2 for all]

In immunocompetent patients, the herpes simplex viruses (cold sores) and the varicella zoster virus (chickenpox and shingles) are the commonest causes. Other examples include cytomegalovirus, HIV, enterovirus, West Nile virus and Japanese encephalitis virus.

There are other causes of encephalitis. In rare cases, it is caused by a bacterial or fungal infection, especially if immunocompromised. Autoimmune examples include Rasmussen's encephalitis, Hashimoto's encephalitis, or acute disseminated encephalomyelitis. No cause can be identified in around half of all cases and it may be a diagnosis of exclusion. A doctor who suspects a diagnosis of encephalitis is legally obliged to report this to the local public health authorities.

9. What do you make of his U&Es?

			Reference range
Sodium	125 mmol/L		136–145 mmol/L
Potassium	5.3 mmol/L		3.6–5.2 mmol/L
Urea	6.5 mmol/L		2.5–6.4 mmol/L
Creatinine	101 μmol/L		80–132 mmol/L

Hyponatraemia can be acute or chronic. The sodium can be low due to syndrome of inappropriate antidiuretic hormone (SIADH) secretion, or related to the chronic liver disease. [1]

10. What treatment measures would you initiate? [2 for all]

This patient has an altered mental status and is at risk of seizure activity. Initial care of seizures is mostly supportive and most seizures are of short duration. Checking airway, breathing and circulation, oxygenation, temperature and blood glucose are important. Intravenous access should be obtained. Prolonged seizures (> 20 minutes) may lead to neurological damage and pharmacological therapy is generally indicated after 5 minutes of fitting.

Lorazepam has a longer half life than diazepam and is preferred. Intranasal midazolam or rectal diazepam are useful if intravenous access is a problem. Repeat benzodiazepine dose at 10 minutes before moving to second-line therapies. These are commonly intravenous phenytoin (20 mg/kg at maximum rate of 1mg/kg per minute) or sodium valproate (10 mg/kg). Optimal dosing of benzodiazepines and second-line drugs should be reviewed before considering third-line agents such as barbiturates, propofol, valproate or levetiracetam.

Intravenous aciclovir should be commenced to treat the likely underlying cause. For treatment of SIADH, refer to page 32.

Data 48

A 55-year-old merchant seaman with diabetes mellitus has been admitted to the medical ward 5 days ago with shortness of breath. He is being treated for suspected PCP and has tested positive for HIV. He has become progressively oliguric and has passed only 50 mL urine in the last 6 hours despite a fluid challenge. Clinically, he is talking in full sentences but feels he is becoming more short of breath.

The medical specialist registrar has requested that the patient be transferred to the intensive therapy unit for renal and respiratory support. It is 22:00 and there are no critical care beds available.

1. What further *clinical* information do you need?
You need observations and fluid balance (given below): [1 for most]
- Blood pressure: 110/45 mmHg
- Heart rate: 100 beats per minute,
- SpO$_2$: 95% (on 50% humidified O$_2$)
- Respiratory rate: 24 beats per minute
- Glasgow Coma Scale (GCS) score: 15
- 2 litres of intravenous normal saline infused in last 4 hours (first intravenous fluids – no fluid balance chart).

2. What is PCP? When does it become a problem?
The type of pneumonia known as PCP (pneumocystis pneumonia) is caused by *Pneumocystis jiroveci* (previously called *Pneumocystis carinii*), which is a type of fungus. This organism is common throughout the population, but does not cause problems in people with healthy immune systems. When a CD4 cell count falls below 200, opportunistic infections are more common and PCP is a classic 'AIDS defining illness'. It often presents with pathological hilar chest X-ray or CT changes, and can be confirmed on broncho alveolar lavage or polymerase chain reaction testing. [2]

3. How is PCP treated? (first line and second line) [2 for all]
Co-trimoxazole (septrin) is the standard first-choice treatment for PCP.
Other options include pentamidine, dapsone, atovaquone, primaquine and clindamycin.
Severe cases may need steroids too.

4. What is septrin? How does it work?
Septrin is a combination of trimethoprim and sulphamethoxazole, which work in synergy by inhibiting bacterial folic acid synthesis. [1]

5. **Take a look at his urea and electroytes (U&Es). Is it appropriate to admit this patient to intensive care with an AIDS-defining illness and two organ (respiratory and renal) failures?**

		Reference range
Sodium	133 mmol/L	136–145 mmol/L
Potassium	5.6 mmol/L	3.6–5.2 mmol/L
Urea	25.0 mmol/L	2.5–6.4 mmol/L
Creatinine	350 µmol/L	80–132 µmol/L

Most would agree that this is an appropriate admission, but the real question is whether this patient actually needs admission at this moment and the answer is, probably, 'No'. HIV infection carries a life expectancy similar to type 2 diabetes mellitus (DM); in the era of highly active antiretroviral treatment (HAART) you shouldn't refuse admission on the basis of HIV diagnosis alone. [2]

6. **Should there be a ceiling of care?**
It would be appropriate to treat aggressively to start with. The short-term prognosis is arguably better than some of the more 'regular' intensive care admissions. [1]

7. **How likely is this patient to survive an intensive care unit stay given his PCP diagnosis?**
For PCP, intensive care unit survival is around 50–70% in the context of HIV. [1]

8. **Why might an HIV-positive patient require intensive care unit admission?** [4 total – 1 each category]
They may require intensive care admission in the case of the following problems:
- Chest: PCP/bacterial pneumonia/tuberculosis (TB)/cytomegalovirus pneumonitis/immune reconstitution inflammatory syndrome
- Central nervous system: lymphoma/progressive multifocal leukoencephalopathy/toxoplasma abscess/meningitis. Consider bacterial, TB or cryptococcus infection
- Sepsis (may be occult and from any focus)
- Cardiac: complications of ischaemic heart disease (IHD)/peripheral vascular disease (PVD) secondary to drug treatment for HIV

9. **What are the potential causes of this man's renal deterioration?**
Potential causes are:
- Pre-renal: hypovolaemia, sepsis [1]
- Renal: chronic diabetic or HIV nephropathy, exposure to nephrotoxins [1]
- Post-renal: exclude obstruction [1]

10. **The medical specialist registrar phones you back to say he thinks he needs 'dialysis'. There are no critical care beds available at present. What are the indications for renal replacement therapy (RRT)? How would you manage this situation?**

The usual indications are hyperkalaemia, volume overload, symptomatic uraemia and acidosis. [1]

In this case, there are no absolute indications for RRT at present.

The lack of a critical care bed is not an uncommon issue faced by consultants. Issues to explore include potentially discharging a 'well' patient from critical care or consider an escalation of beds if local staffing ratios allow. The potential to transfer to another unit is also a possibility that may need to be considered if necessary. [1]

11. **How would you manage this patient if he remains on the ward overnight?** [1]

He should undergo regular monitoring and repeat clinical and biochemical assessment.

A trial of frusemide may be considered to induce diuresis if he is thought to be developing pulmonary oedema, although this is nephrotoxic and its use in the setting of established acute kidney injury is controversial.

Additional information

HIV treatment is a common topic in the examination and candidates should be broadly familiar with treatment options as outlined below.

Highly active antiretroviral treatment (HAART) is the standard treatment, consisting of a combination of at least three drugs that suppress HIV replication. Three drugs are used in order to reduce the likelihood of the virus developing resistance. HAART has the potential both to reduce mortality and morbidity rates among HIV-infected people, and to improve their quality of life.

How do they work?

When HIV infects a cell, reverse transcriptase copies the viral single-stranded RNA genome into a double-stranded viral DNA. The viral DNA is then integrated into the host chromosomal DNA, which then allows host cellular processes, such as transcription and translation to reproduce the virus. Reverse transcriptase inhibitors block reverse transcriptase's enzymatic function and prevent completion of synthesis of the double-stranded viral DNA, thus preventing HIV from multiplying. RTIs can be:

- Nucleoside/nucleotide reverse transcriptase inhibitors, also called nucleoside analogs, such as abacavir (bad in IHD), emtricitabine, and tenofovir. These compete with the 'building blocks' (nucleosides) required to build the viral DNA, causing it to fail.
- Non-nucleoside reverse transcriptase inhibitors (NNRTIs): such as efavirenz, etravirine, and nevirapine. (Risks of Stevens–Johnson syndrome and hepatitis). These interfere directly with the structure of the viral DNA chains.

Other classes of drugs used in HIV infection include:

- Protease inhibitors (PIs), such as atazanavir, darunavir, and ritonavir, which inhibit HIV enzyme required to produce mature infectious viral particles by cleaving structural proteins and enzymes from their precursors. They are potent inhibitors of HIV replication and work synergistically with nucleoside drugs. They are metabolized by cytochrome p450 so have potential for significant drug interactions.
- Entry inhibitors, such as enfuvirtide and maraviroc, which are used after failed triple therapy and stop the HIV virus fusing to the host cell.
- Integrase inhibitors, such as dolutegravir and raltegravir.

The British HIV Association has guidance for starting treatment. This is usually when CD4 counts are stable and below 350 cells/mm^3 or in a new illness and below 200. The goal of treatment must always be to achieve a viral load of less than 50 copies/mL and to achieve this within 4–6 months of starting treatment.

Some medicines are available combined together in one pill. This reduces the number of pills to be taken each day.

Data 49

An 80-year-old lady is admitted to the emergency department following an acute collapse and syncopal episode. She has been unwell for several days with worsening nausea and vomiting and poor oral intake. Her past medical history includes a history of a previous myocardial infarction, heart failure, diabetes and atrial fibrillation. This is her medication list: digoxin 125 µg OD, atenolol 50 mg OD, frusemide 40 mg BD, enalapril 10 mg OD, metformin 500 mg BD and warfarin 5 mg OD. Her laboratory results are as follows:

		Reference range
Sodium	132 mmol/L	136–145 mmol/L
Potassium	3.3 mmol/L	3.6–5.2 mmol/L
Urea	35.8 mmol/L	2.5–6.4 mmol/L
Creatinine	338 µmol/L	80–132 µmol/L
WCC	8.1×10^9/L	$4–11 \times 10^9$/L
Haemoglobin	12.4 g/dL	11.5–16.5 g/dL
Platelets	385×10^9/L	$150–400 \times 10^9$/L
Albumin	30 g/L	35–50 g/L
Total bilirubin	17 µmol/L	3–17 µmol/L
AST	36 IU/L	15–37 IU/L
Alkaline phosphatase	74 IU/L	50–136 IU/L
Glucose	5.1 mmol/L	4.0–5.9 mmol/L
INR	2.1	

1. This is her ECG. Can you comment on this?

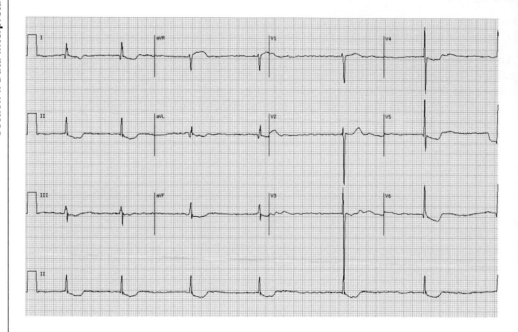

The heart rate is slow (around 40 beats per minute) and the rhythm is irregularly irregular (atrial fibrillation). The axis is normal, as is the width of the QRS complexes. The ST segment has the classical 'scooped out' appearance of digoxin therapy. There is left ventricular hypertrophy by voltage criteria (S wave depth in V1 + tallest R wave height in V5–V6 > 35 mm). [3]

2. What are your concerns here?

This patient has evidence of a severe acute kidney injury (AKI) and has a bradycardia. She may have had an acute cardiac event or be taking too much digoxin and/or beta blocker. The hypokalaemia is probably caused by the loop diuretic and will potentiate the digoxin effects, as will reduced renal clearance. [1]

3. What additional investigations would help confirm your diagnosis?

Raised serum digoxin levels will confirm the diagnosis. [1]

4. What is the mechanism of action of digoxin?

Digoxin acts mainly by binding to the myocardial sodium/potassium ATP-ase pump and inhibiting its action. This inhibition causes an increase in intracellular sodium levels, which are subsequently exchanged for calcium. Increased intracellular calcium increases contractility and also lengthens phase 4 and phase 0 of the cardiac action potential, reducing the heart rate. [1]

5. What ECG disturbances does digoxin toxicity cause?

Increased intracellular calcium causes increased automaticity, classically causing supraventricular tachycardia. Decreased atrioventricular conduction by increasing vagal effects at the atrioventricular node causes slow ventricular responses (atrial tachycardia with block). [1]

6. How would you manage this condition?

Continuous ECG monitoring is essential. [1]

You should carry out treatment of AKI along standard lines including discontinuation of nephrotoxins such as angiotensin-I converting enzyme (ACE-I) and metformin, fluid resuscitation, correction of hypotension and optimization of oxygen delivery. Renal replacement therapy may be necessary in the presence of worsening AKI. [1]

Digoxin-specific antibodies are the mainstay of treatment and bind free digoxin, hence reducing plasma levels. [1]

You should correct any associated electrolyte abnormalities especially hypokalaemia. Digoxin and potassium compete for the same receptor binding site, therefore hypokalaemia potentials digoxin toxicity. [1]

Intravenous glucagon should be considered given the potential for beta-blocker toxicity. [1]

Intravenous atropine may have a role pending definitive management. [1]

You should consider a temporary pacing wire to help manage the severe bradycardia. [1]

7. The patient is admitted to intensive care and appropriate management is commenced. A cardiological review is awaited. She then develops a profound bradycardia with a heart rate of 20 beats per minute unresponsive to atropine, which is associated with haemodynamic compromise. What would you do?

You would commence transcutaneous pacing pending insertion of a temporary pacing wire. [1]

You would consider instituting an adrenaline, isoprenaline or dobutamine infusion. [1]

8. Demonstrate how to perform external pacing on this mannequin.

Commence appropriate sedation as necessary. [1]

Demonstrate appropriate placement of pads either in the anteroposterior or anterolateral position. [1]

Set a target heart rate. [1]

Start with a low current and gradually increase until electrical capture occurs. [1]

Confirm a clinical improvement has occurred as evidenced by a stronger pulse, rise in blood pressure or improvement in conscious level.

Data 50

A 72-year-old male is admitted with acute abdominal pain and vomiting. His abdomen is distended and tender but not peritonitic. He has been assessed by the surgical registrar who has ordered a CT scan of his abdomen. His vital signs are as follows: heart rate 110 beats per minute, blood pressure 100/60 mmHg , respiratory rate 24 breaths per minute, oxygen saturation 93% on room air.

		Reference range
Sodium	140 mmol/L	136–145 mmol/L
Potassium	5.1 mmol/L	3.6–5.2 mmol/L
Urea	8.5 mmol/L	2.5–6.4 mmol/L
Creatinine	140 µmol/L	80–132 µmol/L
Albumin	25 g/L	35–50 g/L
Total bilirubin	31 µmol/L	3–17 µmol/L
AST	160 IU/L	15–37 IU/L
Alkaline phosphatase	140 IU/L	50–136 IU/L
WCC	18.2×10^9/L	$4–11 \times 10^9$/L
Neutrophils	15.1×10^9/L	$2–7.5 \times 10^9$/L
Haemoglobin	13.0 g/dL	11.5–16.5 g/dL
Platelets	290×10^9/L	$150–400 \times 10^9$/L

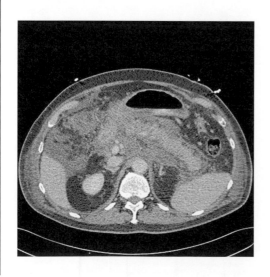

1. What features are visible on this CT scan of the abdomen and what is the likely diagnosis?
The scan shows a swollen, oedematous pancreas with non-enhanced areas of necrosis. [1]
This is indicative of acute pancreatitis. [1]

2. What methods are available to assess the severity of his disease? [2 for most]
There are various scoring systems you can use, e.g.. Ranson's or the Glasgow score. The APACHE and SOFA scoring systems can also be used, although not often for this particular condition. You can use the CT-scan-based scoring to assess severity of necrosis. A clinical assessment and measurement of the degree of organ dysfunction can be justified too.

3. Describe Ranson's criteria. [2 for most]
At admission:
1. Age in years > 55 years
2. White blood cell count > 16,000 cells/mm^3
3. Blood glucose > 11 mmol/L
4. Serum AST > 250 IU/L
5. Serum LDH > 350 IU/L
At 48 hours:
1. Calcium (serum calcium < 2.0 mmol/L)
2. Hematocrit fall > 10%
3. Oxygen (hypoxaemia PO$_2$ < 8 kPa)
4. Blood urea nitrogen increased by 1.8 mmol/L or more after intravenous fluid hydration
5. Base deficit (negative base excess) > 4 mEq/L
6. Sequestration of fluids > 6 L

4. Two days after admission, his condition deteriorates. He exhibits a worsening tachycardia, tachypnoea and hypoxia. Please describe possible reasons for his respiratory deterioration, based on the chest X-ray:

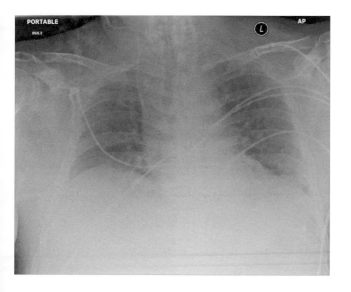

Causes for respiratory deterioration include the following:
- Bilateral effusions [2 for most]
- Atelectasis (from diaphragmatic splinting +/− pain)
- Acute lung injury
- Hospital acquired pneumonia

5. What further information would you like?

Useful information would be a detailed clinical assessment and an arterial blood gas test. [1]

6. These are the results of an arterial blood gas test: On 80% FiO$_2$, pH: 7.30; PaO$_2$: 7.8 kPa; PaCO$_2$: 3.2 kPa. What action will you take now?

The patient should be admitted to critical care. [1]

Oxygen saturation should be maintained > 94%. [1]

Analgesia/chest physiotherapy should be optimized. [1]

Additional respiratory support should be given with continuous positive airway pressure/ intermittent positive pressure ventilation if indicated. [1]

Haemodynamics should be optimized and attention paid to fluid balance. [1]

Intra-abdominal pressures should be measured. [1]

It is important to pay attention to nutrition – ideally using enteral and distal feeding. [1]

7. Would you commence antibiotic treatment?

'Routine' antibiotic prophylaxis is not recommended (there are numerous international guidelines). In patients with infected necrosis, antibiotics known to penetrate pancreatic necrosis may be useful in delaying intervention, thus decreasing morbidity and mortality. Ideally, carry out sampling of necrotic tissue if facilities exist. It is often difficult to distinguish between the inflammatory component and a genuine super-added infective problem. (Talk about the pros and cons of prophylactic antibiotics and antifungals, considering the evidence against routine antibiotics just for prophylaxis). [2]

8. This is a CT scan 3 weeks after initial presentation. What does it show?

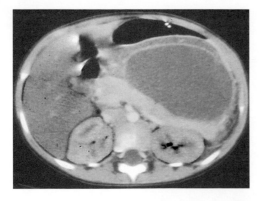

There is a large walled cyst filled with dark material, which seems to arise from the pancreas. This probably represents a large pseudocyst. [1]

9. Does it need treating?

Asymptomatic pancreatic and/or extrapancreatic necrosis and/or pseudocysts do not warrant intervention regardless of size, location and/or extension. In stable patients with infected necrosis, surgical, radiologic and/or endoscopic drainage should be delayed, as mortality is reduced. Consider therapeutic antibiotics for worsening sepsis if this is indicated after cultures have been sent. [1]

Further information

Alternative scoring systems for acute pancreatitis – modified Glasgow score

Assessing the severity of acute pancreatitis

Glasgow prognostic score: (Note PANCREAS acronym)
  a. PaO_2 < 8 kPa (60 mmHg)
  b. Age > 55 years
  c. Neutrophils: (WCC > 15 ×10^9/L
  d. Calcium < 2 mmol/L
  e. Renal function: (Urea > 16 mmol/l)
  f. Enzymes: (AST/ALT > 200 IU/L or LDH > 600 IU/L)
  g. Albumin < 32 g/L
  h. Sugar: (Glucose > 10 mmol/L)

Any three factors means acute severe pancreatitis

Data 51

A 55-year-old adult male is admitted to the intensive care unit with a severe community-acquired pneumonia. He is hypotensive despite fluid resuscitation and commenced on an infusion of noradrenaline. One of your colleagues performs serial blood tests on him and shows you the results: 08:00 sample, serum cortisol 160 nmol/L; 09:00 sample, serum cortisol 300 nmol/L. The table shows the reference ranges.

Reference ranges for blood plasma free cortisol (nmol/L)		
Time	Lower limit	Upper limit
09:00	140	700
Midnight	80	350

1. What test is this? Please comment on the results.
Two serum cortisol samples were assessed. There is a suppressed baseline with a blunted response to stimulation. [1]
This is a synacthen test (or a synthetic adrenocorticotropic hormone (ACTH) test). [1]

2. Tell me about cortisol?
Cortisol is a glucocrticoid steroid hormone, produced by the adrenal gland. [1]
Cortisol's primary functions in the body are:
- Increasing blood sugar through gluconeogenesis
- Aiding in fat, protein, and carbohydrate metabolism
- Anti-inflammatory actions
- Maintaining vascular tone and catecholamine responsiveness [2]

3. What is the normal pattern of serum cortisol levels throughout the day?
Levels usually peak in the morning and fall throughout the day, with some diurnal variation. Levels are stimulated by activity (pattern reverses in night workers) and stress situations. [1]

4. Where does it come from and how is release controlled?
Cortisol is produced in the zona fasciculata of the adrenal cortex. This release is controlled by the hypothalamus. The secretion of corticotropin-releasing hormone (CRH) by the hypothalamus triggers pituitary secretion of ACTH. ACTH is carried by the blood to the adrenal cortex, where it triggers glucocorticoid secretion. There is a negative feedback loop to regulate secretion. [2]

5. What patterns would they expect following a synacthen test for Addison's and pituitary failure?
In pituitary failure, there is no ACTH production and so very little cortisol, but the adrenal glands will still work normally when stimulated by the exogenous ACTH. There will be a low baseline with an exaggerated response. [1]

Addison's disease is the opposite, in that the hypothalamic–pituitary axis is working normally, but there is no target organ response from the adrenal glands. There will be low baseline cortisol (with high endogenous ACTH if you measured it) with very little response to synacthen. [1]

6. What are the commonest causes for primary adrenal failure?

- Autoimmune (Addison's disease) [2]
- Infiltration with tumour or tuberculosis
- Meningococcal sepsis (Waterhouse–Friedrichsen syndrome) or ischaemia

7. What other tests could be done to establish the cause of the low cortisol? [2]

Measure the serum hormone levels: ACTH, aldosterone and renin.

Check the serum electrolytes influenced by cortisol: potassium and sodium.

Consider obtaining a CT scan of the adrenal glands.

Test for 21-hydroxylase autoantibodies to diagnose adrenal insufficiency of autoimmune origin, as this represents more than 90 percent of all cases in a Western population.

8. What is secondary and tertiary adrenal failure?

Secondary adrenal failure is a result of absent ACTH secretion resulting from primary pituitary pathology (tumours, surgery, Sheehan's syndrome) or a suppression of secretion secondary to the exogenous administration of steroids. Tertiary adrenal failure occurs as a result of failure of hypothalamic CRH secretion. [1]

9. Under what circumstances do we opt to replace cortisol in critical care practice? [2]

We might consider replacing cortisol:

- In cases of long-term steroid dosing (long term considered > 7.5 mg for > 3 months)
- Where these is genuine pituitary or adrenal failure
- Following high-dose steroid treatment

Another potential indication for its use is in the treatment of vasopressor refractory septic shock.

10. Should we do more synacthen tests in intensive care?

No. The adrenal axis often malfunctions in the critically ill resulting in a wide variation in cortisol levels with no clear thresholds or cut-off values to identify those with and without adrenal insufficiency. Responses to ACTH do not identify patients who would benefit from steroid administration. [1]

11. What do you make of these blood results from a different patient?

	Result	Reference
TSH	2.9 mIU/L	0.2–4.0 mIU/L
free T4	16 pmol/L	10–20 pmol/L
total T3	0.6 nmol/L	0.9–2.5 nmol/L

There is a low total T3 level associated with normal T4 and thyroid-stimulating hormone (TSH) levels. The absence of a high TSH level excludes primary hypothyroidism. This pattern would fit a sick euthyroid syndrome, often seen in starvation or critical illness. [2]

12. What causes sick euthyroid syndrome? [1]

There is dysregulation (or abnormal adaptation) of thyrotropic feedback control where the levels of T3 and/or T4 are abnormal, but the thyroid gland does not appear to be dysfunctional. Most active T3 is produced outside the thyroid by peripheral conversion from T4. This mechanism also fails, leading to normal or sometimes high T4, but low T3. T4 can confusingly be low sometimes due to low levels of its transport proteins in critical illness.

Another definition of sick euthyroid syndrome is where abnormal thyroid function tests occur in the setting of a non-thyroidal illness, without pre-existing hypothalamic–pituitary and thyroid gland dysfunction. After recovery from the non-thyroidal illness, the thyroid function test result abnormalities should be completely reversible. Pre-existing thyroid disease makes this condition very difficult to diagnose and treat and expert help should be requested.

Data 52

A young man presents to the emergency department having fallen off a ladder. He is conscious and haemodynamically stable although he does have a suspected pelvic fracture. His blood results are as follows:

		Reference range
WCC	12.0×10^9/L	$4–11 \times 10^9$/L
Haemoglobin	13.0 g/dL	11.5–16.5 g/dL
Platelets	345×10^9/L	$150–400 \times 10^9$/L
INR	1.1	
APTT	62 seconds	28–38 seconds

1. **What could be the cause of the activated partial thromboplastin time (APTT) being prolonged in this case?**

Prolonged APTT may indicate:
- The use of heparin (or contamination of the sample) [1]
- The presence of antiphospholipid antibody/lupus anticoagulant (which paradoxically increases the tendency to thrombosis) or presence of specific antibodies against coagulation factors [1]
- Coagulation factor deficiency (e.g. haemophilia) [1]
- Coagulopathy of trauma/disseminated intravascular coagulation (although isolated APTT rise here make this unlikely) [1]

2. **Which clotting factors does the APTT test depend on and which pathway does it test?**

The APTT tests the intrinsic pathway of coagulation including factors XII, XI, IX, VIII, V, II and I. [1]
This pathway is initiated by the interaction of Factor XII with a negatively charged surface. [1]

3. **What other laboratory tests relating to coagulation could you ask for?**
- Fibrinogen and fibrin degradation products (FDP) [1]
- Point of care tests – for example TEG [1]

4. **What is a TEG test?**

A thromboelastography (TEG) test is a haemostatic assay that measures the global visco-elastic properties of whole blood clot formation. The interaction of platelets with the coagulation cascade (aggregation, clot strengthening, fibrin cross linking and fibrinolysis) is demonstrated. Importantly, TEG does not necessarily correlate with blood tests such as INR, APTT and platelet count, which can be poor predictors of bleeding and thrombosis. [1]

5. **This is a TEG test. What do these four patterns represent?** [4 for all]

1. Normal R, K, MA and angle
2. Anticoagulants, factor deficiency, haemophilia:
   • R and K prolonged, MA and angle decreased
3. Platelet blockers, thrombocytopaenia, platelet dysfunction
   • R normal, K prolonged, MA decreased
4. Fibrinolysis
   • R normal, MA decreasing

6. **This gentleman now becomes haemodynamically unstable with increasing tachycardia and a fall in blood pressure. What principles would you use to manage this situation?**

Check airway, breathing and circulation, including cervical spine protection, and assess for life-threatening injuries. [1]

Control haemorrhage and stabilize fractures. [1]

Include here identifying other sources of haemorrhage. [1]

Trigger a massive transfusion pathway and administer blood products 4:4:1 (red blood cells/fresh frozen plasma/platelets). [1]

Avoid hypothermia/acidosis. [1]

Give tranexamic acid (see the CRASH 2 trial: *Lancet* 2011; 377(9771): 1096–1101)) [1]

7. **How would you define a massive transfusion? (Any reasonable definition may be accepted.)**

A massive transfusion may be defined as follows: in adult patients, a transfusion of half of one blood volume in 4 hours, or more than one blood volume in 24 hours (adult blood volume is approx 70 mL/kg). [1]

TEG explanation

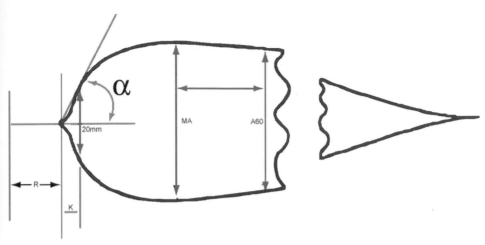

For the colour version, please refer to the plate section. In some formats this figure will only appear in black and white.

Specific parameters represent the three phases of the cell-based model of haemostasis: initiation, amplification and propagation

- R value = reaction time(s); time of latency from start of test to initial fibrin formation – clot initiation
- K = kinetics(s); time taken to achieve a certain level of clot strength – clot amplification
- alpha = angle (slope between R and K); measures the speed at which fibrin builds up and cross linking takes place, assesses the rate of clot formation
- TMA = time to maximum amplitude(s)
- MA = maximum amplitude (mm); represents the ultimate strength of the fibrin clot
- A30/A60 = amplitude at 30/60 minutes
- LY30 – defined as percentage of clot that has lysed at 30 minutes.

Data 53

These are blood results taken from a 50-year-old male alcoholic who has been admitted in a comatose state after having been found collapsed in the street. No other corroborative history is currently available.

		Reference range
Sodium	137 mmol/L	136–145 mmol/L
Potassium	5.0 mmol/L	3.6–5.2 mmol/L
Urea	10.4 mmol/L	2.5–6.4 mmol/L
Creatinine	155 µmol/L	80–132 µmol/L
Chloride	104 mmol/L	95–105 mmol/L
Albumin	21 g/L	35–50 g/L
Total bilirubin	18 µmol/L	3–17 g/L
AST	40 IU/L	15–37 IU/L
Alkaline phosphatase	85 IU/L	50–136 IU/L
INR	1.3	
APTT	35 seconds	28–38 seconds
FiO_2	0.21	
pH	7.05	7.35–7.45
pO_2	11.5 kPa	10.0–14 kPa
pCO_2	2.5 kPa	4.4–5.9 kPa
Bicarbonate	12.0 mmol/L	22–28 mmol/L
BE	−15.1 mEq/L	−2–(+2) mEq/L
Lactate	16.2 mmol/L	0–2 mmol/L

Electrocardiogram (ECG): normal sinus rhythm; chest X-ray: normal; CT brain scan: normal.

1. What other investigations would you want?
- Sepsis screen [1]
- Salicylate and paracetamol levels and urine toxicology screen [1]
- Blood alcohol plus ethylene glycol levels (difficult to measure and usually have to be sent away to a tertiary laboratory) [1]
- Blood glucose and ketones [1]

2. **Tell me how you would calculate the anion gap. Is it raised?**

Anion gap $= (Na^+ + K^+) - (Cl^- + HCO_3^-) = (137 + 5.0) - (104 + 12) = 26$

Normal ranges depend on measurement but are widely considered as 8 to 16 mEq/L plasma when not including $[K^+]$ and from 10 to 20 mEq/L otherwise. This patient has a raised anion gap metabolic acidosis.   [1]

3. **What else would you like to measure in the plasma?**
It would be useful to measure the serum osmolality, both calculated and measured.   [1]

4. **What is the osmolar gap and how would you calculate this?**

Osmolar gap $=$ measured serum osmolality $-$ calculated osmolality
Calculated osmolality $= 2 \times [Na \; mmol/L] + [glucose \; mmol/L] + [urea \; mmol/L]$ [1]
An osmolar gap > 10 is abnormal.   [1]

4. **The osmolar gap is raised. What is the likely diagnosis?**
This is likely a case of ethanol or ethylene glycol poisoning.   [2]

5. **What are the clinical features that can be seen with ethylene glycol poisoning?**
- *Neurological*:   [1]
  - Initial symptoms can be very similar to acute alcohol intoxication with inebriation, slurred speech, euphoria and drowsiness, which may progress to cerebral oedema, convulsions and coma
  - A delayed neurologic presentation occurring long after ingestion has been described and is characterized by weakness and cranial nerve palsies
- *Cardiovascular*:   [1]
  - Dysrhythmias, myocardial depression, hypotension and heart failure. Severe metabolic acidosis is often a feature
- *Renal*:   [1]
  - Acute tubular necrosis occurs as a result of the direct toxic effects of glycolate on renal tubules and the deposition of calcium oxalate crystals within renal tubules

6. **Why is the lactate so high?**
This is commonly a laboratory error. Glycolate can cause large artifactual elevations in plasma L-lactate measurements with common analysers, leading to the potential for misdiagnosis of a severe lactic acidosis in ethylene glycol poisoning.
However, there may be coexistent tissue hypoperfusion, which causes the high lactate. [2]

7. **What specific treatment would you institute?**
In addition to general supportive critical care, metabolic acidosis may necessitate the administration of bicarbonate and (mechanical) hyperventilation.   [1]
Specific antidotes include ethanol or fomepizole.   [1]
These are competitive antagonists with a high affinity for the enzyme alcohol dehydrogenase and delay metabolism until the ethylene glycol is eliminated naturally or via dialysis.   [1]
Haemodialysis could be considered to aid elimination.   [1]

8. **Who could you discuss the case with to obtain further advice?**
The National Poisons Information Service should be able to offer useful advice.   [1]

Data 54

Introduction

As for chest X-rays, you need to have a systematic approach for describing and interpreting ECGs, both for examinations and in clinical practice. Your system should be flexible enough to adapt to various clinical settings and examination styles.

It doesn't matter too much what system you use but it should be clear to the examiner that you are demonstrating a logical system. Once you have done this, the examiner will usually direct you towards describing the relevant pathology or diagnosis, although this may vary a little with examiner styles.

A detailed description of how to interpret the ECG is beyond the scope of this book, but a suggested approach is to describe the ECG as follows:

1. Heart rate (beats per minute (bpm), state atrial and ventricular rates if different)
2. Rhythm (sinus, atrial flutter, etc.)
3. QRS axis in frontal plane
4. Work through the PQRST complex:
   a. P-wave morphology
   b. PR interval (from beginning of P to beginning of QRS)
   c. Q waves present?
   d. QRS duration (width of most representative QRS)
   e. T-wave morphology
   f. ST segment changes
   g. QT interval (from beginning of QRS to end of T)
5. Look for patterns such as left ventricular hypertrophy (LVH), adjacent ischaemic segments, conduction blocks
6. Summarize and interpret

The ECG electrodes or 'leads' are presented in a pattern. Leads II, III and aVF 'look' at the inferior part of the heart, I and aVL look laterally, and the precordial leads V1 to V6 work their way from the right ventricle, across the septum to the left ventricle.

1. A 50-year-old lady presents with gradual onset shortness of breath.

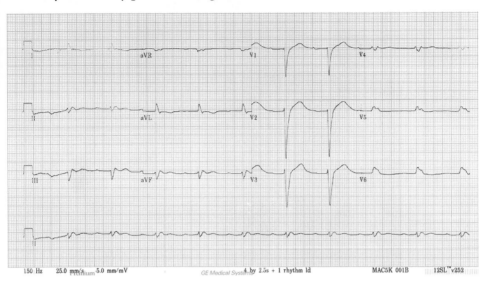

The ECG shows sinus rhythm with a rate of 60 bpm and first-degree atrioventricular (AV) block. The axis is –30 degrees and the QTc is prolonged at 600 milliseconds. There is left bundle branch block (LBBB). Multiple conduction abnormalities are often ischaemic in origin, which may explain this lady's symptoms.

2. A 65-year-old woman presents with an acutely ischaemic distal leg.

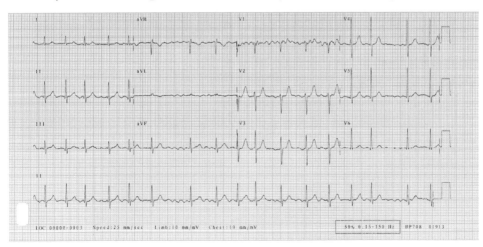

The rhythm is irregularly irregular suggesting atrial fibrillation (there are a few organized P waves seen in the rhythm strip so flutter/fibrillation is reasonable) with a ventricular rate of around 100 bmp. QRS axis is 30 degrees with no other significant abnormalities present. The atria do not contract in AF and so clots can form due to blood stasis. This may be a cardiac source of emboli to her leg.

3. A 55-year-old man presents with palpitations.

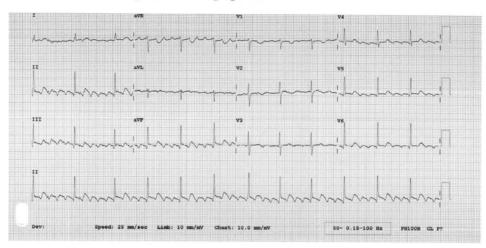

The atrial rate is 300 and the ventricular rate is 75, meaning atrial flutter with a predominantly 4:1 block. The axis is normal. There may be some ST elevation in the inferior leads but this is difficult to interpret with the superimposed flutter waves and clinical correlation is required.

4. A 76-year-old man presents during a spontaneous breathing trial from ventilation.

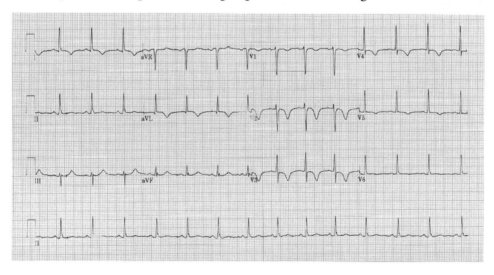

Rate is 80 bpm with normal sinus rhythm and a normal axis. There is widespread T inversion in I, aVL and across the precordial leads. This implies anterolateral ischaemia and should be compared with previous ECGs. If new, the weaning attempt should be abandoned and the ischaemia investigated and treated.

5. An 84-year-old man presents to the emergency department with syncopal episodes.

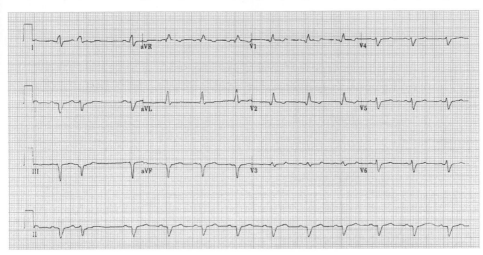

The ECG is in normal sinus rhythm with a normal PR interval. The rate is 70 bpm and the axis is leftward at –80 degrees. There is right bundle branch block (RBBB) and a left anterior fascicular block (LAFB) making a bifascicular block. The conduction abnormalities are significant given the history and he is only one fascicle away from complete heart block.

6. An elderly lady has collapsed in the supermarket. She presents with low blood pressure in the emergency department.

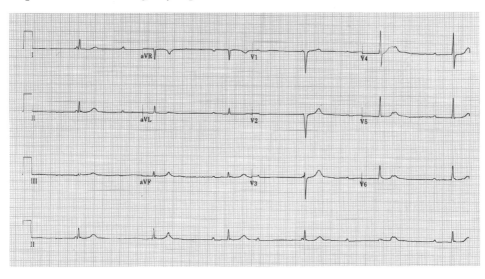

The ECG has a ventricular rate of around 35 bpm. There are P waves present but they bear no consistent relationship to the QRS complexes, implying complete heart block. There are septal Q waves (V1 to V3) and the QRS complex is narrow. This would suggest a junctional bradycardia escape rhythm. If she is symptomatic, then she is likely to need pacing, although a trial of positive chronotrope may be indicated.

7. A 66-year-old coal miner presents with progressive shortness of breath.

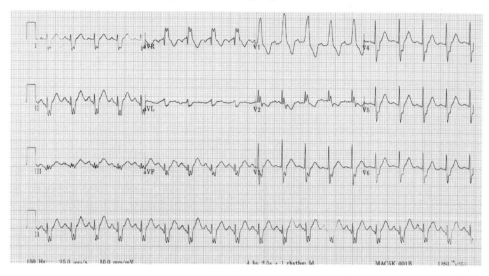

There is a sinus tachycardia with a ventricular rate of 110 bpm. The axis is rightwards (200 degrees) and the QRS complex is widened. There is a positive R wave in V1 so this is RBBB. There are no abnormal P waves. This could represent cor pulmonale.

8. An elderly lady from India presents. She has had symptoms of heart failure for many years.

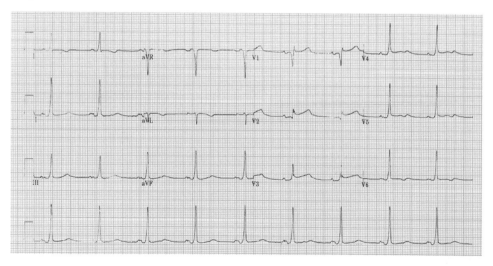

The ECG has a rate of 60 bpm in sinus rhythm. The QRS axis is normal at 45 degrees. The P waves are abnormal: 0.12 seconds long with a characteristic 'm' shape (p mitrale). This implies an enlarged left atrium. The QRS complexes are normal but there are biphasic T waves seen laterally in V4–V6 which may imply ischaemia. The lady may have mitral valve disease, but against this is the fact that she is not in atrial fibrillation. Clinical assessment is required, along with an echocardiogram.

9. **A young man is brought in with rapid tachycardias. The emergency department specialist registrar was about to give some adenosine but he spontaneously reverted and this is his ECG.**

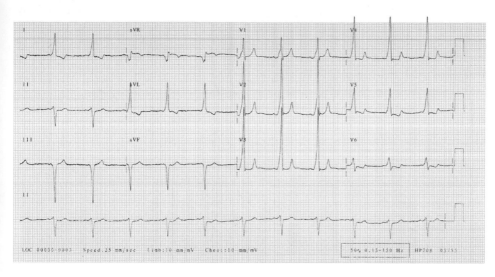

The ECG shows normal sinus rhythm at a rate of 70 bpm and a leftward axis. The PR interval is short and there is a slurred upstroke into the QRS complex. This delta wave is pathognomic of Wolff–Parkinson–White syndrome (type A due to the positive R wave in V1 – secondary to a left atrioventricular accessory pathway (the Bundle of Kent). Because of the electrophysiologic differences between AV nodal tissue and an accessory pathway, adenosine or other drugs for heart rate control may actually worsen symptoms and promote malignant ventricular tachycardias involving the accessory pathway. Treatment of choice for tachycardias is procainamide (or amiodarone) or electrical cardioversion.

10. **A 66-year-old man presents on the intensive care unit, whose blood pressure keeps suddenly dropping for a few seconds, and then it returns.**

The ECG has two pacing spikes: one where the P wave should be and the second at the start of the (abnormal) QRS complex. This is a dual-chamber pacemaker, rendering the rest of the ECG interpretation almost impossible. On the rhythm strip, each beat is paced both at the atrial and ventricular level, implying that the pacemaker was working effectively, at least whilst the ECG was taken. The history is suggestive of loss of electrical capture or pacemaker malfunction and a rhythm strip from the intensive care unit monitor should be examined. A pacemaker check is an easy non-invasive procedure to perform, but requires specialist software and equipment, bespoke to the type and manufacturer of the device.

Data 55

Introduction

You need to have a systematic approach for describing and interpreting chest X-rays both for examinations and in clinical practice. This ensures no important structures or pathologies are ignored. Your system should be flexible enough to adapt to various clinical settings.

It doesn't matter what system you use but it should be clear to the examiner that you are demonstrating a logical system. Once you have done this, the examiner will usually direct you towards describing the relevant pathology or diagnosis, although this may vary a little with examiner styles.

Always start by commenting on the name and identifiers of the patient (usually removed and anonymized for examinations) and a comment on the adequacy of the image. This means that it should show all of the relevant field and be adequately penetrated and exposed. This is usually the case for an examination. The mnemonic PIER can help:

- P – position – supine/anterior–posterior (AP)/posterior–anterior (PA)/lateral
- I – inspiration – at least 10 posterior ribs for an adequate inspiration
- E – exposure – good lung detail and an outline of the spinal column
- R – rotation – compare clavicles with midline structures such as vertebrae

For example:

> This is a PA (it will state this on the film) or AP/mobile chest film of the patient referred to in the question. There is adequate exposure and penetration of the field and structures of interest and the image is not significantly rotated. Working sequentially through the film, I can see . . .

If the examiner is directing you to move through this introduction and logical assessment, you can move to stating what the most obvious abnormality is. Always try and link the image to the clinical information provided. If there are multiple lines and monitoring devices in place, mention these, for example:

> There is an appropriately positioned right internal jugular central line, an appropriately positioned endotracheal tube siting above the carina, an oesphageal Doppler probe and multiple ECG electrodes, implying that the patient is likely critically ill.

Here are some suggested logical systems in brief:

1. **Anatomical approach**
    1. Trachea/bronchi
    2. Hilar structures
    3. Lung zones
    4. Pleura
    5. Lung lobes/fissures
    6. Costophrenic angles
    7. Diaphragm
    8. Heart
    9. Mediastinum
    10. Soft tissues
    11. Bones

2. **ABCDE**
   A. Airways
   B. Bones
   C. Cardiac (heart and vessels)
   D. Diaphragm
   E. Everything else! (lungs and lines)
3. **ABCDEFGHI**
   A. Assessment of quality – PIER
   B. Bones and soft tissues – fractures, foreign bodies, subcutaneous air
   C. Cardiac size (< 50% of the chest diameter on PA films and < 60% on AP films, shape, prosthetic valves)
   D. Diaphragms – right usually higher. Can you see it all? Any air underneath?
   E. Effusions – clear costophrenic angles?
   F. Check lung fields for infiltrates (interstitial versus alveolar), masses, consolidation, air bronchograms, pneumothoraces and vascular markings
   G. Great vessels – aortic knuckle and aorta and pulmonary truck
   H. Hila and mediastinum – masses, widening, tracheal deviation
   I. Impression – putting it all together

For brevity, the answers given below represent the significant abnormalities only and do not comment on all of the systematic elements described above.

1. An abdominal plain film from a patient who isn't absorbing their feed.

It shows centrally located multiple dilated loops of gas-filled bowel. *Valvulae conniventes* are visible (small bowel) but there is also large bowel gas and gas in the stomach. There is no obvious blockage implying likely ileus but this would need clinical correlation.

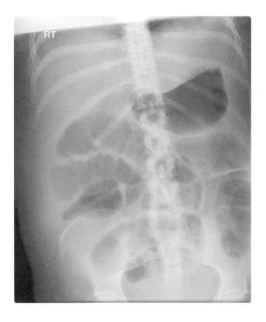

2. **A chest X-ray of a 50-year-old man with chronic breathlessness admitted to the intensive care unit for respiratory support.**

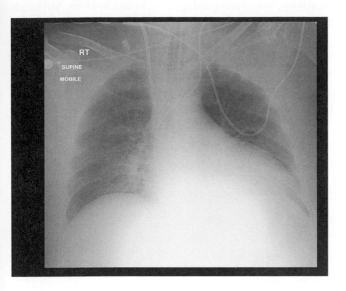

The patient is intubated and there is a right internal jugular central venous catheter (RIJ CVC) and a left internal jugular pulmonary artery catheter (LIJ PAC). Allowing for the AP projection, the heart is grossly enlarged and there is pulmonary oedema. Chronic heart failure or a cardiomyopathy are likely from the chest X-ray and clues from the invasive monitoring.

3. **A contrast-enhanced CT brain scan from a 45-year-old homeless man who presents with seizures.**

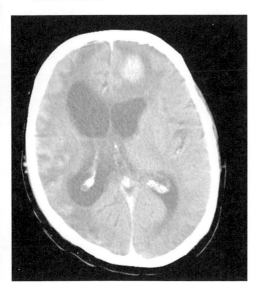

This image shows a left frontal enhancing mass (white) with surrounding grey oedema. There is effacement (squashing) of the sulci on both sides and mid-line deviation to the right. Both lateral ventricles appear large, suggesting a degree of hydrocephalus, although the left is effaced somewhat by the mass. This could represent a tumour or abscess.

4. **A non-contrast CT brain scan from a man presenting with a severe headache and sudden collapse.**

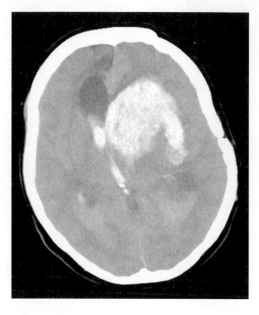

This un-enhanced CT shows a large intracerebral haemorrhage (white) in the left fronto-parietal region. There is surrounding oedema, effacement of the sulci and left lateral ventricle and deviation of the mid-line to the right. The appearances and history are consistent with a posterior communicating artery aneurysm rupture.

5. **A chest X-ray from an elderly man who is recovering from a pneumococcal pneumonia. He has been ventilated for 2 weeks.**

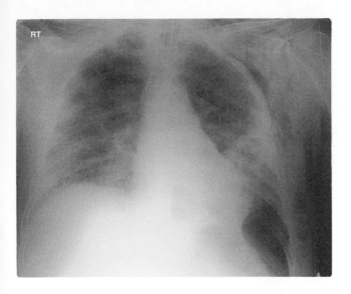

An endotracheal tube (ETT) and LIJ CVC are *in situ*. Both mid and lower zones of the lung fields are filled with patchy opacities with loss of the costophrenic angle on the right, implying a pleural effusion. The most obvious abnormality is the dark shadow at the left lung base. This appears to be loculated and extending down beyond the base of the chest film, with consolidated lung above. This likely represents a loculated pneumothorax. A better exposed chest X-ray and perhaps an ultrasound scan would help here.

6. **A chest X-ray of a 66-year-old woman who becomes short of breath after an episode of chest pain and requires resuscitation.**

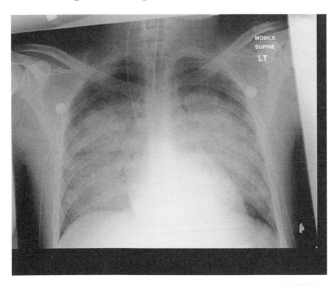

There is an ETT and RIJ CVC *in situ*. There is upper-zone vessel enlargement implying pulmonary venous hypertension with bilateral increased perihilar lung markings (bats wings). Septal (Kerley B) lines are visible but no pleural effusions or cardiomegaly. This is likely acute pulmonary oedema.

7. **A chest X-ray from a 54-year-old man whose gas exchange gets worse after an attempted chest drain.**

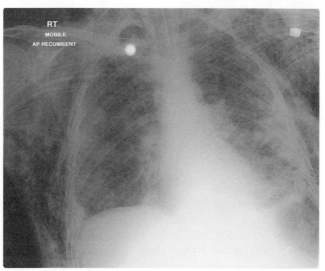

There is an ETT, LIJ CVC, nasogastric (NG) tube with the tip in the stomach and, significantly, a left basal chest drain. There still appears to be a residual pneumothorax. There is a 'cotton-wool' appearance over the chest and in the visible soft tissues implying extensive bilateral surgical emphysema. There is also bilateral perihilar opacification.

8. **A chest X-ray of an elderly lady about to go to theatre for a laparotomy.**

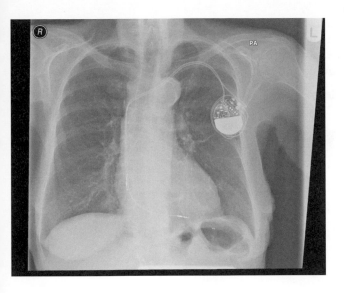

The substance of the chest X-ray is unremarkable. There is a dual-chamber cardiac pacemaker *in situ*. The leads terminate in right atrial appendage and right ventricular apex. There are no shock coils and so this is not an intra-cardiac defibrillator (ICD). You should make sure that the theatre team are aware of the pacemaker, including the settings, last check and the reason for insertion (i.e. what will happen if it stops working!)

9. **Image intensifier printout of an elderly female patient who has just come back from interventional radiology.**

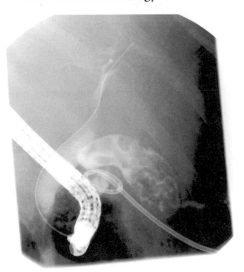

This is endoscopic retrograde cholangiopancreatography (ERCP). The side-angled endoscope has been passed into the duodenum and the biliary tree has been catheterized via the ampulla of Vater. Contrast is seen in the hepatic ducts. There is contrast in the gall bladder with multiple filling defects, implying likely gall stones. There is a small amount of contrast outside the biliary system, which has a pig-tailed drain adjacent to it. There is the possibility of peritoneal gas, although this could just be from the endoscopic procedure with the duodenum overlying. The drain was likely placed for a previously noted gall-bladder perforation and this is the follow up ERCP.

10. **A chest X-ray from an elderly steel worker who has been ventilated on the intensive care unit for 3 weeks.**

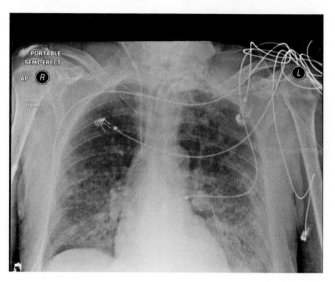

This is a portable film that doesn't catch the left lung base. A tracheostomy tube, RIJ CVC, fine-bore NG tube and ECG monitoring are *in situ*. There is an extensive reticular pattern seen throughout both lungs most marked in the mid and lower zones. There is also fluid noted in the horizontal fissure. The lung parenchymal appearances are suggestive of fibrosis.

11. **MRI scan from a 62-year-old male driver involved in a high-speed road traffic accident.**

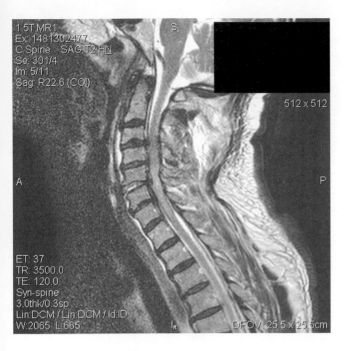

This is a sagittal MR slice through the cervical spine. C4, C5 and C6 are abnormal and the body of C6 appears to have fractured. There is anterior oedema. There is loss of the bright white cerebral spinal fluid space around the spinal cord and the cord itself appears to have sustained a contusion with the darker area visible around C4. This shows a cervical spine fracture with cervical cord involvement.

12. A plain CT scan from a 55-year-old woman who collapsed at work.

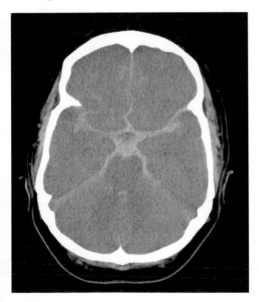

The dense white material in the basal cisterns and fissures in a five-pointed-star pattern is due to acute bleeding into the subarachnoid space.

13 A chest X-ray taken from a woman who has been ventilated for 10 days.

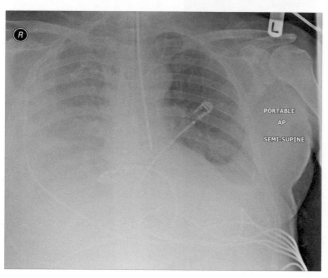

An ETT, LIJ CVC and oesophageal Doppler probe are *in situ*, along with ECG monitoring. The right hemithorax is opacified with loss of the diaphragm. The mediastinum is not displaced. This likely represents a large pleural effusion. There is a smaller effusion on the left.

14. A hypoxic middle-aged female patient who was recently intubated. There is not much improvement in gas exchange.

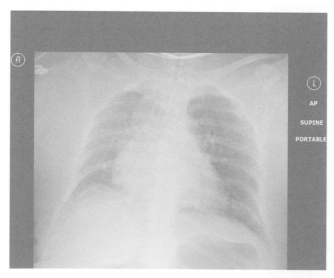

This portable film shows an ETT with the tip sited quite far down the right main bronchus. There is volume loss on the right with the mediastinum deviated to the right. The tip may be beyond the bronchus intermedius as there appears to be little air in the right upper lobe.

15. A CT scan of the thorax of a hypoxic, obese, middle-aged female patient.

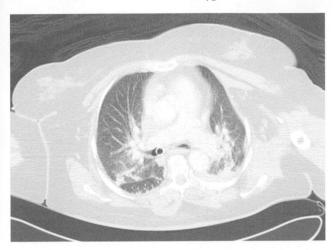

This rather embarrassing CT scan shows the ETT placed in the right main bronchus. There is associated volume loss and basal atelectasis of the left lung.

16. The CT scan of a young lady with refractory hypoxia despite aggressive ventilation.

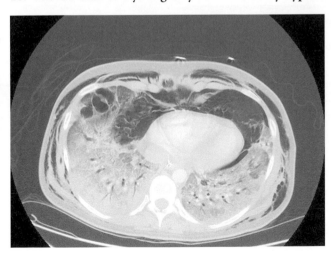

Bilateral dependent grossly consolidated lungs with air bronchograms and traction bronchiectasis are visible. There are bilateral anterior pneumothoraces and air is also seen in the soft tissues. The artefact in the oesophagus is probably a Doppler probe.

17. A chest X-ray taken on a young man after theatre following a deceleration injury.

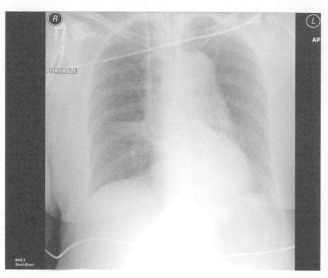

A chest X-ray shows an ETT and RIJ CVC. There is a thoracic aortic stent that extends from the aortic arch into the descending aorta. This was presumably placed endovascularly to treat a traumatic dissection.

18. A chest X-ray from a patient with pneumonia and acute leukaemia.

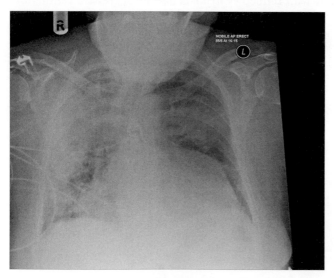

This mobile film shows extensive patchy opacification throughout the right lung field, most marked in the right upper zone. There is volume loss and the trachea is deviated to the right. This probably represents a right upper lobe pneumonia. The heart contour is enlarged and abnormal. Without any clear signs of heart failure in the visible left lung, a pericardial effusion should be considered.

19. A 60-year-old man with long-standing back problems presents with shortness of breath.

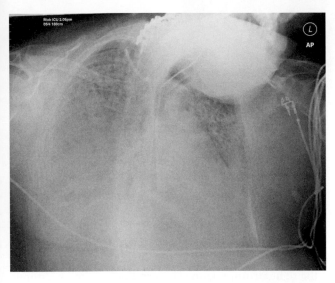

There are several bony abnormalities: the visible thoracic spine appears like a long tube. The intervertebral discs have ossified giving the 'bamboo spine' appearance associated with ankylosing spondylitis. There is an internal upper thoracic–cervical fixation device. The lung fields have bilateral patchy opacification with some smooth grey 'ground glass' regions (mid zone right, lower zone left). There is peri-bronchial cuffing implying extravasated lung water and the distribution of the oedema implied a global alveolar capillary leak, such as that seen in an acute lung injury (rather than the more dependent pattern in heart failure).

20. This 53-year-old male patient had refractory hypoxia. Can you describe the X-ray and tell me what has happened?

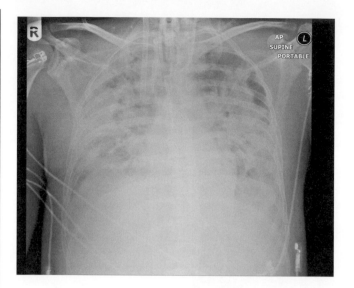

There is a tracheostomy, NG tube, ECG monitoring and a LIJ CVC *in situ*. There is a large cannula in the RIJ with the tip in the right atrium region. There is another similar cannula arising from below the diaphragm, presumably in the inferior vena cava (IVC). The tip ends near the right heart. The lung fields are small and there are widespread patchy opacities throughout with air bronchograms. There may be a left upper zone pneumothorax. The lung appearances are consistent with ARDS. The vascular devices are extra corporeal membrane oxygenation (ECMO) cannulae – one dual lumen catheter in the RIJ and an additional 'sump' to drain venous blood via the femoral approach to the IVC.

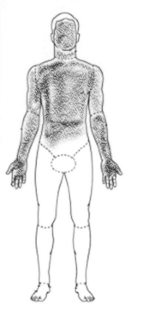 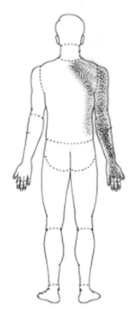

ANTERIOR POSTERIOR

Data 4.1 Burns assessment completed

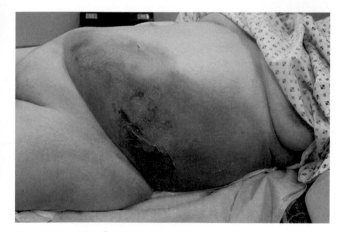

Data 7 Necrotizing fasciitis

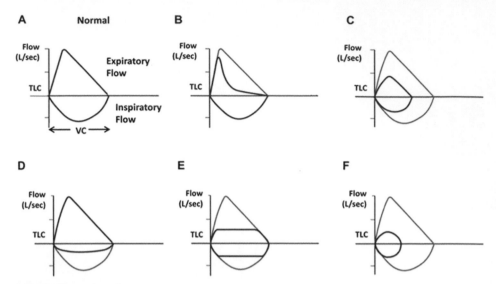

Data 12 Flow volume loops

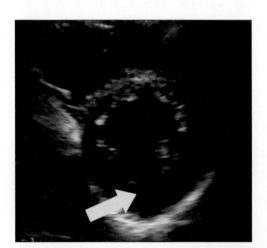

Data 21.2 Parasternal short axis view, arrow points to inferior wall

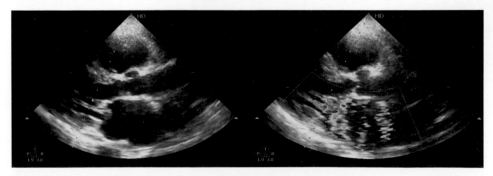

Data 21.3 Parasternal long axis view, mitral valve prolapse

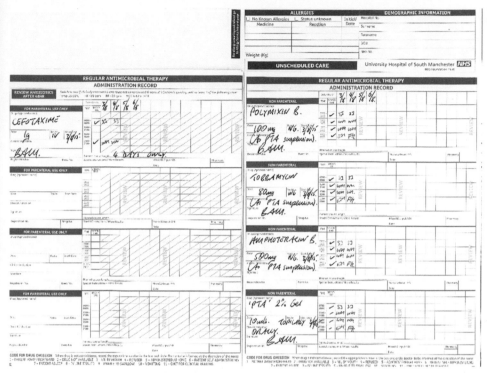

Data 31 SDD drug chart

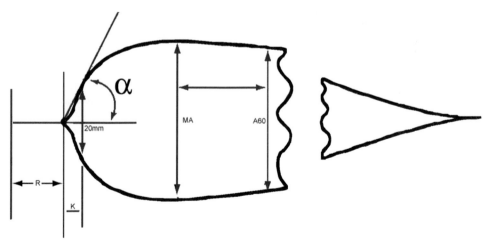

Data 52.2 TEG

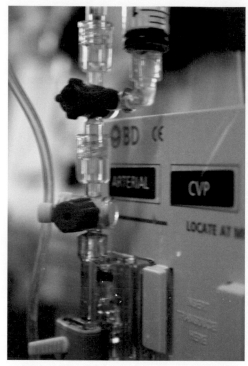

Equipment 1.1 Art line transducer

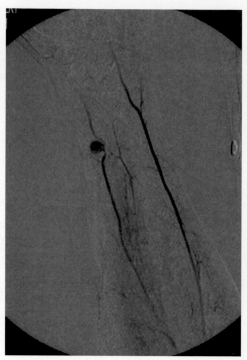

Equipment 1.3 DSA of radial artery aneurysm

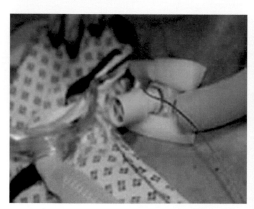

Equipment 2 Speaking valve *in situ*

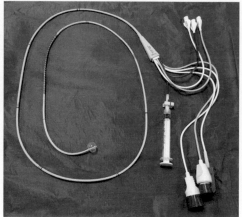

Equipment 5.1 PAC

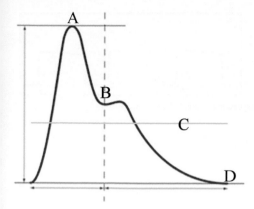

Equipment 8.1 Arterial waveforms 1

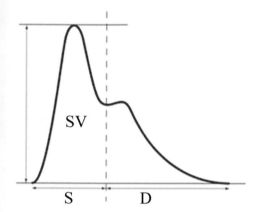

Equipment 8.2 Arterial waveforms 2

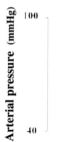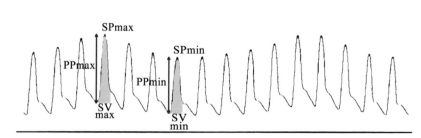

Equipment 8.4 Arterial waveforms 4

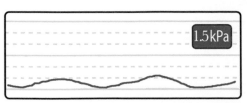

Equipment 10 Spinal needles

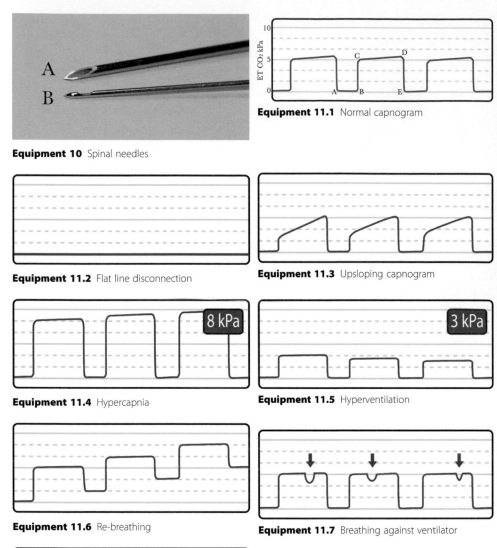

Equipment 11.1 Normal capnogram

Equipment 11.2 Flat line disconnection

Equipment 11.3 Upsloping capnogram

8 kPa

Equipment 11.4 Hypercapnia

3 kPa

Equipment 11.5 Hyperventilation

Equipment 11.6 Re-breathing

Equipment 11.7 Breathing against ventilator

Equipment 11.8 Cardiac vibrations

Equipment 11.9 Oesophageal intubation

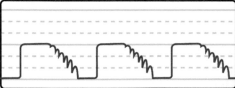

1.5kPa

Equipment 11.10 CPR capnogram

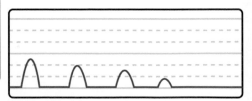

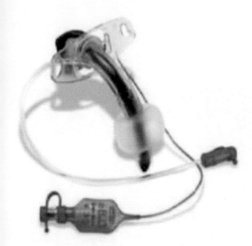

Equipment 13.1 SGS trachy tube

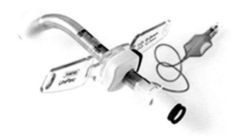

Equipment 13.2 Adjustable-length (Flange) trachy tube

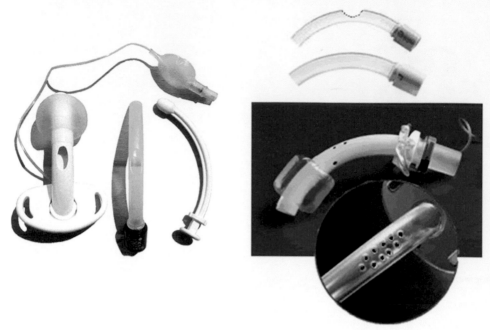

Equipment 13.3 Fenestrated trachy tube

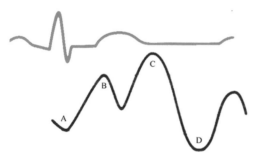

Equipment 16 IABP pressure trace (BMs)

Equipment 1

1. What is this equipment and what are the key components?

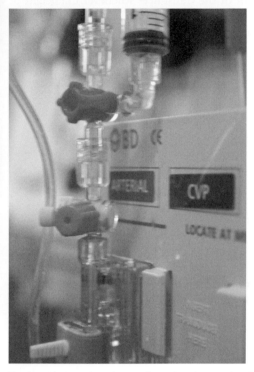

For the colour version, please refer to the plate section. In some formats this figure will only appear in black and white.

This is an arterial line transducer system. It consists of a 500 mL bag of pressurized fluid (saline or heparinized saline), stiff, non-compliant tubing, a transducer system and a cable connecting it to the monitor.   [2]

2. How does an arterial transducer work?

Basically, this is a system designed to convert mechanical signals into electrical signals. Changes in pressure are transmitted via fluid-filled rigid tubing to the pressure transducer, which contains an inbuilt diaphragm. Movement of the diaphragm results in changes in resistance in an inbuilt strain gauge converting the signal into an electric one via a wheat stone bridge. This electric signal is then transmitted via a cable to a microprocessor where it is further amplified and processed through Fourier analysis and displayed on a monitor.   [2]

3. **A student nurse has just learnt how to set this up and is about to connect it to the patient. What further advice would you give her?**

The arterial line needs to be calibrated to atmospheric pressure. The zero level chosen is usually the 4th intercostal space in the mid axillary line (which corresponds to the right atrium). [1]

To zero the transducer, turn the stopcock off to the patient and open to the air. It is important to remember to change the height of the transducer whenever the height of the bed is altered. [2]

Remember to ensure that the transducer system is free from bubbles prior to connecting to the patient. [1]

4. **Look at these arterial line waveforms. The left-hand image (A) is normal. What do you think is going on with the other two? Why is this important to detect?**

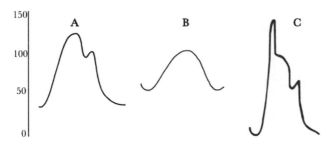

The centre image (B) is an over-damped arterial waveform. It results in erroneous measurement of blood pressure (BP) with under-reading of systolic BP and over-reading of diastolic BP and can lead to incorrect therapeutic interventions. The right-hand image (C) is under-damped and the exaggerated waveform can lead to overestimation of systolic and underestimation of diastolic blood pressure. [2]

5. **Can you explain to the nurse what resonance and damping mean?**

The measurement system has a natural resonant frequency. This relates to how fast the system vibrates in response to a pressure signal. To be responsive to changes in pressure, the system's natural resonance should match that of the signal being measured as closely as possible. This means that if an arterial pressure changes at a (heart) rate of 120 beats per minute, the natural resonant frequency should be around 2 times per second (2 Hertz). However, the system would go on vibrating unless it was stopped. This requires damping and leads to a decrease in the amplitude of oscillations due to a loss of energy in the system. Optimal damping stops the resonance in the system from distorting and amplifying the signal too much, whilst maintaining a rapid enough response. [2]

6. **What factors can contribute to over-damping?** [1 for most]

Causes of over-damping include:

- The presence of air bubbles
- The use of tubing that is long, too narrow or compliant
- Kinks in the arterial line
- Blood clots
- Vasospasm

7. Is dextrose appropriate as a flush solution?

No. There have been several reported cases of inadvertent hypoglycaemia and even death occurring after inappropriate treatment of hyperglycaemia caused by sampling a dextrose containing arterial line solution. [2]

8. A patient complains of pain in his hand 6 hours after insertion of a radial arterial line. What action would you take?

Take a history to assess the character of the pain and associated symptoms such as numbness or paraesthesia.

Perform an examination, checking for the colour of the digits, cap refill, sensation and movement. [1 for both]

If in doubt take the arterial line out. Continue close monitoring for improvement of symptoms and signs after device removal. If there is no improvement, an urgent vascular opinion should be sought. [2]

9. Look at this picture. What is the investigation and what complication has occurred?

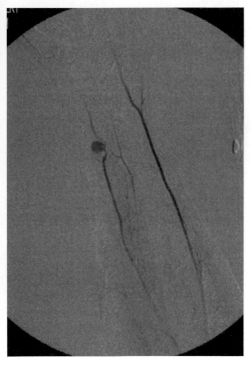

For the colour version, please refer to the plate section. In some formats this figure will only appear in black and white.

This is a digital subtraction angiogram (DSA) of the forearm. It shows the radial and ulnar arteries. This is a distal radial pseudo-aneurysm which has developed after an arterial line insertion. This is a bulge in the artery wall. [2]

179

Equipment 2

A 55-year-old man required a temporary percutaneous tracheostomy 10 days ago to facilitate weaning from mechanical ventilation. He had an acute lung injury following smoke inhalation in a house fire 3 weeks ago. He is now breathing spontaneously on 20 cmH$_2$O pressure support ventilation, with a continuous positive airway pressure of 6 cmH$_2$0 and an FiO$_2$ of 40%. He is alert and co-operative and otherwise well.

1. How would you define weaning delay and failure? [2 for both]

There are various definitions, including failing more than three spontaneous breathing trials (SBTs) and requiring more than seven days of mechanical ventilation following the first SBT.

The need for ventilatory support for more than 2 weeks in the absence of any non-respiratory factor preventing weaning is weaning delay, with 3 weeks being failure.

2. What proportion of intensive care patients that are ventilated will prove difficult to wean?

The difficult-to-wean patient represents around 6% of the intensive care population, but consumes a third of resources. Such patients experience increased morbidity and mortality.[1]

3. What factors can contribute to weaning delay? [6 for all]

- *Metabolic*:
  - . Metabolic alkalosis, usually from diuretics or from chronically raised CO$_2$
  - . Hypophosphataemia
  - . Hypothyroidism
- *Respiratory*:
  - . Latent respiratory disease, unmasked by the critical illness
  - . Unresolved primary respiratory pathology (or new infection)
  - . Pleural effusion
- *Cardiac*:
  - . Pre-existing and intensive care acquired cardiac dysfunction
  - . Weaning-induced ventricular dysfunction (changes in intrathoracic pressures and by increases in sympathetic tone as respiratory support is reduced)
- *Fluid distribution*:
  - . Renal dysfunction and hypoalbuminaemia can contribute to oedema of tissues and lungs
- *Airway*:
  - . A degree of airway-device misplacement or unknown airway pathology can significantly increase the work of breathing
- *Central nervous system*:
  - . Depression
  - . Delirium
  - . Latent or new neuropathies or myopathies

4. Assuming we exclude or correct these factors, what are the principles behind successful weaning? [2]

There are various strategies but principles include:

- Adequate rest – higher support pressures, especially at night. Reduce support during the day
- Gradual reductions in support
- 'Sprints' where support is rapidly reduced (or removed) for shorter periods
- Down-sizing of the tracheostomy tube or changing for a fenestrated tube
- Periods of cuff deflation

5. What is this? How does it work?

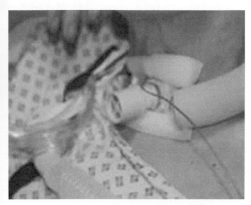

For the colour version, please refer to the plate section. In some formats this figure will only appear in black and white.

This is a Passey–Muir speaking valve attached to a cuffed tracheostomy tube (pilot tube is visible). This is a one-way valve that is attached to the ventilator-end of the tracheostomy tube. During inspiration, the valve is open but it closes during expiration. Gas cannot exit via the lumen of the tracheostomy tube. This forces exhaled gas around the tube and up through the larynx. [2]

6. Are there any safety precautions that need to be taken with it? [2]

It must never be used with a cuff-inflated tracheostomy tube as this would lead to complete asphyxia. Even a cuffed tube with the cuff deflated must be used carefully as the risk is that someone will inflate the cuff. It is most safely used with un-cuffed or fenestrated tubes. Use caution if excess secretions.

It increases the resistance to expiration and therefore the work of breathing.

7. Other than speaking valves, how else can we communicate with patients like this?

Lip reading is difficult and not all patients can write easily whilst critically ill. Communication boards can be simple or electronic, involving touchpads. [1]

8. Why do you get high cuff pressures? [2 for all]

High cuff pressures can cause mucosal ischaemia and should be limited to 20–25 cmH$_2$O. A small tube in a large calibre trachea will need a lot of gas (and likely pressure) to create an adequate seal.

High airway pressures delivered will need a cuff pressure at least as high in order to prevent a gas leak.

A faulty device or leak from the pilot balloon/cuff system can require constant addition of air to the cuff.

Finally, a poorly positioned or ill-fitting tube may need cuff hyperinflation to overcome these problems. High cuff pressure should always be investigated.

9. How do you introduce oral feed in a tracheostomized patient? [2]

This is a balance of alertness, laryngeal sensation and function, cough and swallowing. Some patients can swallow with the cuff inflated but most need to have the cuff deflated and therefore be well enough to tolerate this.

A detailed assessment by speech and language therapists can help ensure that oral diet is commenced safely.

Equipment 3

1. This is a picture of the bronchial tree. Can you tell me what the labels represent?

[8 for all]

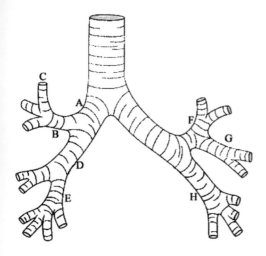

A. Right main bronchus
B. Right upper lobar bronchus
C. Apical segment of right upper lobe
D. Bronchus intermedius
E. Right lower lobe bronchus
F. Left upper lobe bronchus
G. Lingular division
H. Left lower lobe bronchus

2. Can you outline some indications for which you would consider bronchoscopy.

[4 for all]

- Diagnostic uses include:
  - The aspiration of sputum or cytology samples for microbiological or pathological analysis
  - Visualization of bronchial tree in airway trauma, for burns or if a lung lesion (tumour or inhaled foreign body) is suspected
  - Aspiration can be assisted by first instilling small volumes (typically 20 mL) of saline during a bronchial wash (BW) or a more formal broncho-alveolar lavage (BAL)
- Therapeutic uses:
  - BW may also be used as a therapeutic manoeuvre for lobar collapse via the removal of mucus plugs or secretions

3. Talk me through a BAL

BAL involves instilling 50–200 mL of saline into a target lung segment. As much saline as possible is aspirated back through the bronchoscope and collected by placing a sample chamber between the bronchoscope suction port and the wall suction. Samples are often for cytological or immunological analysis, although larger volumes of saline can be used to try and remove particulate matter and debris or in therapeutic lavages such as following smoke inhalation with contamination of the bronchial tree. [2]

3 What are the main risks associated with bronchoscopy? [2 for all]
The main risks include:
- Hypoxia, difficulty with ventilation, V/Q mismatch, bronchospasm
- Hyperinflation/air trapping/barotraum/pneumothorax
- Miscellaneous – high intracranial pressure/bleeding/tachycardia/hypertension

4. How would you minimize these risks?
The risks can be minimized with:
- Pre-oxygenation [1]
- Adequate monitoring (oxygen saturation/capnography) [1]
- An appropriate-sized endotracheal tube [1]
- Appropriate sedation and/or muscle relaxant [1]
- Minimizing duration (allow time in between for recruitment)/limiting amount of saline used for washouts [1 for any]

Equipment 4

A patient is admitted to the intensive care unit sedated and ventilated as they did not wake up following a witnessed, out-of-hospital cardiac arrest and return of spontaneous circulation (ROSC). Your colleagues have commenced external cooling.

1. How does therapeutic hypothermia work?

Therapeutic hypothermia probably works by decreasing the metabolic rate of the brain, by decreasing the release of harmful molecules such as free radicals, by stabilizing cell membranes and by other poorly understood mechanisms. [1]

2. What are the inclusion criteria to cool these sorts of patients? [2 for all]

Therapeutic hypothermia is an option for these patients, although recent evidence from the Targeted Temperature Management (TTM) trial (*NEJM* 2013; 369: 2197–2206) has led to debate about how low to cool patients. Avoidance of pyrexia is paramount. Patients who meet the following criteria are eligible for therapeutic hypothermia:

1. Cardiac arrest with return of cardiac output
2. < 15 minutes between collapse and first attempt at resuscitation
3. < 60 minutes from collapse to ROSC
4. Comatose and requiring respiratory support
5. Able to maintain a systolic blood pressure > 90 mmHg (even if vasopressors are required)

3. Are there any exclusions? [2 for all]

Exclusions to use of therapeutic hypothermia include the following:

1. Coma due to a primary neurological event
2. Medical co-morbidities that would otherwise preclude intensive care unit referral
3. Severe sepsis
4. Bleeding or coagulopathy are relative contraindications (cooling causes coagulopathy)
5. Actively bleeding (N.B. thrombolysis is **not** a contraindication)
6. Core temperature < 30 °C at presentation
7. Prolonged hypotension or hypoxia (secondary brain injury)

If a patient is awake and appropriate enough not to require intubation, these patients do not need hypothermic neuroprotection.

4. Should we perform a CT brain scan? [2 for justification and opinion]

A CT brain is not mandatory for comatose patients following cardiac arrest. The history and clinical features may indicate a primary cardiac event that led to the arrest and subsequent hypoxic brain injury (explaining the neurological picture). If there is any doubt or suspicion that a primary neurological event may have occurred then a CT brain scan should be undertaken. The sequence of CT or percutaneous coronary intervention (PCI or 'angioplasty') should be agreed with senior clinicians, usually at consultant level. A primary cerebral event or bleed may cause secondary cardiac arrest and if clinical features or history suggest a primary neurological event, then treatment will be different (avoiding anticoagulation, neurosurgical opinion). An early CT scan will not help in establishing the severity of a hypoxic brain injury and should not delay PCI, cooling or definitive critical care.

5. What equipment options are available to cool this patient? [3 for all]

There are a variety of methods available, including cold intravenous fluids, external cooling and invasive body cavity or vascular cooling.

The simplest method of initiating cooling is infusing cold crystalloid at 4 °C (Hartmann's or normal saline). A stunned myocardium following ROSC may not tolerate aggressive volume loading. The use of 250 mL boluses with clinical reassessment is recommended.

External cutaneous devices range from chilled pads or ice packs through to systems that circulate cooled fluid to a target temperature.

Invasive vascular devices are less portable and can lead to insertion complications but offer definitive cooling.

6. How do we monitor temperature in cooled patients?

We monitor the core body temperature (e.g. oesophageal, rectal, bladder, pulmonary artery catheter). [1]

7. What complications can arise from cooling? [2 for all]

Hypothermia may cause arterial spasm and complicate arterial line insertion.

Pressure sores can occur with vasoconstricted hypoperfused skin. Skin care and good nursing care is essential, especially where skin is in contact with cooling devices.

Bradycardia is a possible complication. If it is severe (i.e. less than 25–30 beats per minute) then consider treatment with antimuscarinics (not always effective in the cooled patients) or B-agonists, or consider raising the target temperature.

Sedative requirements will be less when the brain is cooled down.

Shivering can be a further complication.

Hypokalaemia can develop with cooling. Although systemic cooling has a likely cardioprotective effect, low potassium levels can contribute to dysrhythmias, especially in the post cardiac arrest patient.

8. Tell me about electrolyte and arterial blood gas changes with cooling. [2 for all]

When blood is cooled, carbon dioxide becomes more soluble. This reduces the measured $PaCO_2$ by about 4.5% per °C.

Haemoglobin accepts more hydrogen ions when cooled meaning the pH rises (more alkaline).

There are two ways of interpreting the samples: without correction (alpha-stat management) or by the addition of CO_2 to normalize pH (pH-stat management).

Potassium, magnesium and phosphate move intracellularly during hypothermia, lowering serum concentrations. On re-warming, the extracellular shift of anions may lead to increasing plasma concentrations.

9. Is shivering a problem?

Even if the patient is not obviously shivering then so called 'micro-shivering' can still occur.

Shivering is undesirable as it makes the patient more difficult to cool, and will increase their oxygen demand. [1]

10. How do you manage shivering? [2 for all]

Shivering usually occurs during cooling and is less of a problem once target temperatures are achieved (if the target is below 35 °C).

Boluses or increasing infusions of sedation can be effective.

Warming the extremities with gloves or socks can reduce shivering.

Pethidine lowers the threshold for shivering and can be given in boluses of 25 mg if the use of a neuromuscular blockade is to be avoided.

A neuromuscular blockade is most likely to be needed during the initial cooling-down phase and during the warming-up phase. It may not be required whilst the patient is stable between 32 and 34 °C. Using the peripheral nerve stimulator, the 'train of four' should be kept between 1 and 2. If there is a concern about possible seizure activity then remember that this might be masked by an infusion of neuromuscular blockade.

11. How do we manage re-warming with a surface cooling device? [1 for most]

Re-warming should begin 24 hours after cooling commenced.

The ideal rate of re-warming is between 0.2 and 0.5°C per hour i.e. it should take around 6–8 hours to get from 33°C to 36°C.

Patients with brain injuries can become hyperthermic and may need to be actively cooled again. Rebound hyperthermia is a recognized phenomenon in these patients (perhaps in around one third).

A neuromuscular block may be required during the re-warming phase, to avoid the increased metabolic demand caused by shivering.

Watch for hypotension as the patient vasodilates. Intravenous fluids may be required.

Stop any potassium infusions during re-warming as the potassium level is likely to rise.

12. Can enteral feeding be continued during cooling?

Nasogastric feeding can be safely undertaken during periods of hypothermia. There is probably a reduction in gastric motility with hypothermia, so have a lower threshold for suspending feed until normothermic. [1]

Equipment 5

1. What is this piece of equipment?

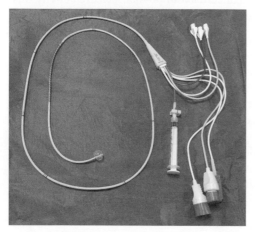

For the colour version, please refer to the plate section. In some formats this figure will only appear in black and white.

This is a pulmonary artery (Swan–Ganz) catheter. [1]

2. What is it used for?

It is used for measurement of cardiac output using the principle of thermodilution. A bolus of cold fluid (10 mL cold saline) is injected and the subsequent change in temperature is measured through a thermistor at the distal end. Cardiac output is inversely proportional to the change in temperature over time (Stewart–Hamilton equation). [2]

It is used for direct measurement of right-sided heart pressures and pulmonary capillary wedge pressure (as an indicator of left ventricular end diastolic pressure) and mixed venous oxygen saturation. [2]

Indirect variables measured include systemic and pulmonary vascular resistance. [1]

1. Look at this waveform. Can you describe events taking place at points A, B, C and D?

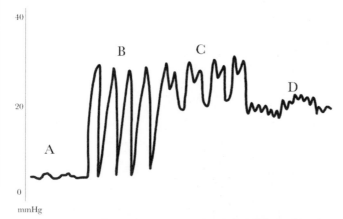

A. This is a central venous pressure trace reflecting right atrial pressure (0–6 mmHg) [1]
B. This is a trace of the catheter in the right ventricle (systolic pressure 15–30 mmHg, diastolic pressure 2–8 mmHg) [1]
C. This is a trace obtained from the pulmonary artery (systolic pressure 15–30 mmHg, diastolic pressure 8–15 mmHg) [1]
D. This is a pulmonary capillary wedge pressure trace (8–15 mmHg) [1]

4. Tell me about some complications associated with the use of a pulmonary artery catheter?

There are complications related to cannulation, e.g. pneumothorax or arterial puncture and bleeding. [1]

There are complications related to the passage of the catheter, such as arrhythmias, pulmonary infarction, valvular damage, malposition and knotting of the catheter. [2]

There can be late complications, e.g. infection. [1]

5. Why do you think its use is dwindling?

There are several reasons for this: [3]

- The evidence base shows no real evidence of a benefit in terms of mortality reduction (e.g. the PAC-Man trial; *Lancet* 2005; 366(9484): 472–477)
- It is an invasive technique with a not insignificant risk of complications/harms associated with its use
- There are other alternatives to measure cardiac output using less invasive monitors and echocardiography
- Medical and nursing staff are increasingly unfamiliar with its use

6. This is the chest X-ray of a patient with cardiogenic shock. What is going on?

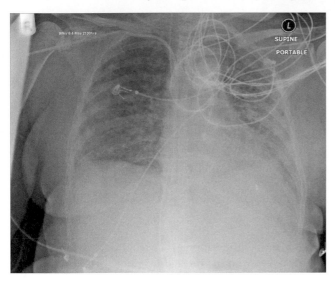

This lady has an endotracheal tube (ETT) *in situ* and a mass of ECG monitoring. There is a right subclavian line which is assumed to be a pulmonary artery catheter (PAC) due to its length and ultimate tip position in the right ventricle. The PAC loops down into the inferior vena cava before returning to the heart and should be removed. The left hemidiaphragm is elevated (a nasogastric tube is seen in the stomach to help identify this) and there is increased opacity at the left lung base. [3]

Equipment 6

1. This is the chest X-ray of a patient in critical care. Can you comment?

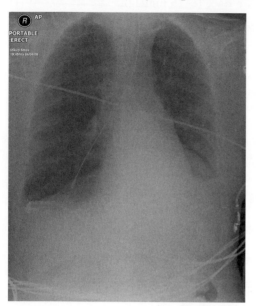

It is an erect, portable, anterior–posterior chest film of a patient with ECG monitoring attached. The nasogastric tube (NG) is clearly seen entering the right main bronchus and passing into the right lung base. There is left basal volume loss, loss of costophrenic angle and likely left basal pleural effusion. [2]

2. Do you know of any guidelines related to the insertion of NG tubes?
A National Patient Safety Agency (NPSA) alert in 2011 highlighted the issue of detecting the inadvertent placement of NG tubes. Recommendations made include: [2]
(a) Using pH strips as a first line of confirmation with a pH of aspirated fluid between 1 and 5.5 to exclude pulmonary placement
(b) Radiological confirmation if you are unable to confirm with pH testing; NG tubes should be radio opaque along their entire length
There may be a role for testing using bedside electromagnetic devices but at present these are only advised for second-line testing.
Ongoing management includes the regular documentation of the length of the tube and pH checks before each use. Further confirmation with pH testing or radiological confirmation may be needed if migration of the NG tube is suspected. [1]

3. What are the indications for placing an NG tube? [2 for all]
NICE guidelines suggest placing an NG tube in patients who are malnourished or who are at risk of malnourishment and
(a) have inadequate or unsafe oral intake
(b) have a functional gastro-intestinal (GI) tract with no contraindications to enteral feeding

4. Can you name some potential contraindications? [3 for all]

Potential contraindications are the following:

- Base of skull fracture
- Oesophageal varices
- Coagulopathy
- Recent nasal surgery

5. Demonstrate how you would go about inserting an NG tube in this mannequin (if present, or describe if not). [3 for a good description]

1. Explain and take verbal consent.
2. Wear non-sterile gloves.
3. Estimate the distance of insertion – from ear lobe to nose and to xiphisternum.
4. Sit the patient up and choose an appropriate nostril (you could ask the patient to sniff).
5. Ensure adequate lubrication.
6. Insert along the floor of the nose until it is visible in pharynx.
7. If cooperative, ask the patient to swallow to aid passage (sips of water if it is safe to do so) and advance gently until the appropriate level is reached.
8. Stop and withdraw tube if the patient is distressed or coughing.
9. Secure in place, confirm the position with pH testing or an X-ray and document.

6. Feeding via a misplaced NG tube is a 'never event'. Do you know of any other never events in critical care? [max. 3]

Some never events applicable to critical care include:

- Wrong site procedures
- Wrongly prepared high-risk injectable medication
- Maladministration of potassium-containing solutions
- Wrong route of drug administration
- Maladministration of insulin
- Failure to monitor and respond to oxygen saturations
- Chest or neck entrapment in bedrails
- Scalding of patients
- Transfusion of incompatible blood products
- Retained foreign body post procedure

7. **Can you describe these two X-rays taken on the same patient contemporaneously?**

[2 for both]

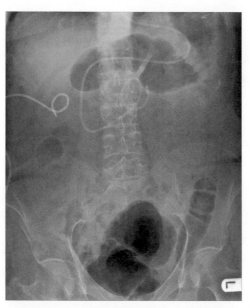

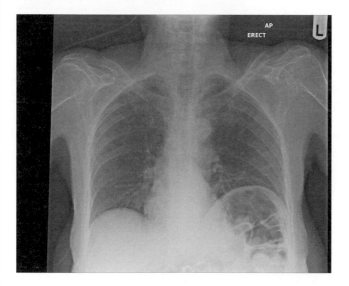

The abdominal film shows some gaseous distension in loops of small bowel and gas in the rectum. There is a trans-gastric tube that terminates in the proximal jejunum. There is a pig-tailed drain in the right flank which is probably a nephrostomy. This is a naso-jejunal (NJ) tube.

The chest film shows the NJ tube again in the oesophagus and looping round in what appears to be a distended stomach. The chest is otherwise unremarkable. These images would be consistent with a recently inserted NJ tube with the upper GI tract gas likely related to endoscopic insertion.

7. When would you consider inserting NJ tubes and what are the methods of insertion?

[2 for both]

They are indicated for post pyloric feeding in patients with severe reflux or delayed gastric motility.

They can be inserted blindly, for example by advancing the tube by 10 cm every hour once in the stomach up to the 100-cm mark. Passage is aided by the administration of prokinetics. Devices are available with magnets, tracking systems and special coatings to help with peristaltic self-propulsion beyond the pylorus. NJ tubes can also be inserted under endoscopic or fluoroscopic guidance.

Equipment 7

Consider a patient in respiratory failure due to pneumonia admitted to your intensive care unit. There is a history suggestive of chronic obstructive pulmonary disease (COPD).

1. **If they are hypoxic despite standard oxygen therapies delivered by open face-mask, what treatment options are there for respiratory support, and which would you choose?**

Invasive mechanical ventilation is probably the best choice for *de novo* hypoxaemic respiratory failure and non-invasive ventilation (NIV) is more likely to fail in hypoxaemic patients. [1]

NIV is the mode of choice in acute respiratory failure due to COPD exacerbations, acute cardiogenic pulmonary oedema, and hypoxaemic failure in immunocompromised patients. [1]

NIV improves outcome of patients who succeed, by avoiding intubation, but it may worsen outcome by delaying intubation in those having failed NIV. This is difficult to predict, but decide and justify your answer. With a history of COPD, a trial of NIV to start with is reasonable. [1]

2. **What are the disadvantages of invasive ventilation in this setting?** [2 for all]

There may be intubation peri-procedural problems (airway management, cardiac).

There is a risk of laryngeal or tracheal injury from the endotracheal tube (ETT).

Host defences are impaired (cough, mucociliary transport) and there is potential for developing ventilator-associated pneumonia.

Ventilator-associated complications may also include barotrauma, air trapping and dynamic hyperinflation, patient–ventilator dyssynchrony and respiratory muscle dysfunction.

Invasive ventilation requires sedation.

3. **What are the physiological effects of NIV?** [2 for all]

The respiratory mechanics are improved: this generates larger tidal volumes, reduces atelectasis and aids recruitment and also reduces the work of breathing.

There are cardiac effects: decreased left ventricular afterload, and reduced left and right ventricular preload.

4. **Are there any non-invasive alternatives that you are aware of other than face-mask-delivered NIV to treat the hypoxia?** [2 for both]

Alternative interfaces include full head hoods or nasal masks.

A high-flow nasal cannula (HFNC) may also be considered, especially in the context of type 1 respiratory failure.

5. **What are the current potential uses for an HFNC in intensive care?** [3 for all]

- *De novo* type 1 respiratory failure e.g. secondary to pneumonia (FLORALI study, *NEJM* 2015; 372: 2185–96)
- Post-operative respiratory failure
- During bronchoscopy
- Pre (and per) oxygenation prior to (or during) intubation
- Post-extubation respiratory distress

6. What does the equipment to deliver oxygen via an HFNC consist of?
The equipment consists of an air/oxygen blender, an active heated humidifier, a single heated circuit and the nasal cannula itself. Air/oxygen is delivered at high flows into the upper airways and generates a degree of continuous positive airway pressure by offering resistance to expired air. [2]

7. What sorts of gas flow rates are delivered to the patient?
Flow rates of up to 70 L/min are possible. [1]

8. What sort of inspiratory flow rates can a patient with respiratory failure generate?
Inspiratory flow of patients varies widely in a range from 30 to more than 100 L/min. [1]

9. What relevance does this have to the breathing systems used to deliver oxygen?
Conventional devices will have oxygen flows < 15 L/min leading to entrainment of room air, resulting in variable and lower-than-expected FiO_2. HFNC systems generate higher flow rates, exceeding the patient's peak inspiratory flow rate in most cases, resulting in a stable FiO_2 that is closer to that intended to be delivered. [1]

10. What do we mean by the term 'dead space?'
Dead space is the part of the respiratory tract that does not contribute to gas exchange. This can be *anatomical* (upper airways, trachea, proximal bronchi), where there are no alveoli, or *physiological*, where there is a ventilation/perfusion (V/Q) mismatch. [1]

11. What are the effects of a closed NIV face-mask and HFNC on dead space?
NIV interfaces increase anatomical dead space but lung recruitment and reversal of atelectasis may reduce physiological dead space by improving V/Q mismatch. HFNC decreases physiological dead space by lung recruitment without additional anatomical dead space. [1]

12. Are there any effects of HFNC on arterial concentration of carbon dioxide?
CPAP pressures are relatively low with HFNC compared with closed systems, but are adequate enough to increase lung volume or recruit collapsed alveoli. This will increase tidal volume and hence minute volume, aiding elimination of CO_2. Carbon dioxide is also 'washed out' in the anatomical dead space by the high flows. [1]

Equipment 8

Candidates are shown the arterial waveform.

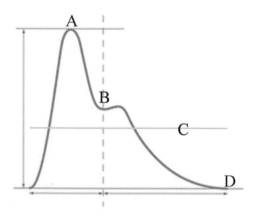

For the colour version, please refer to the plate section. In some formats this figure will only appear in black and white.

1. Can you tell me what the points ABCD are? [1 for all]
A. Peak systolic pressure
B. Dicrotic notch (*incisura*): drop in pressure when the aortic valve closes; followed by the dicrotic wave of reflected aortic flow
C. Mean arterial blood pressure
D. Diastolic blood pressure

2. Where do systole and diastole occur? [1 for both]
The answers are marked as S and D on the image below.

3. What represents the stroke volume?
This is the area marked SV on the image below. [1]

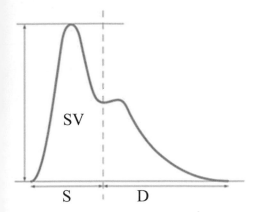

For the colour version, please refer to the plate section. In some formats this figure will only appear in black and white.

4. If the contractility increased, how would the waveform change?
The slope of the upstroke of the systolic waveform would get steeper if the contractility increased.

5. Why there is a cyclical change in the measured arterial pressure in this second waveform below?

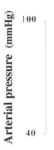
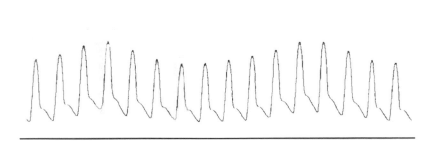

Time (seconds)

The cardiac output (Q) can be affected significantly by the phase of respiration; intrathoracic pressure changes influence diastolic filling and therefore Q. This is especially important during mechanical ventilation where Q can vary by up to 50% across a single respiratory cycle. [1]

6. With relation to the diagram, draw on where you would measure the following
- Stroke volume variation (with respiration) [SVmax to SVmin] [1]
- Pulse pressure variation [PPmax to PPmin] [1]
- Systolic pressure variation [SPmax to SPmin] [1]

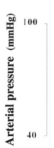

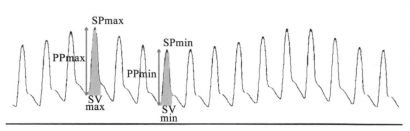

Time (seconds)

For the colour version, please refer to the plate section. In some formats this figure will only appear in black and white.

7. With regard to pulse pressure variation – what is actually being measured?

What is actually being measured are the respiratory changes in arterial pressure in a mechanically ventilated patient. The pulse pressure (PP; systolic minus diastolic pressure) is minimal (PPmin) three heart beats after its maximal value (PPmax) in the figure above. [1]

The respiratory changes in pulse pressure (ΔPP) can be calculated as the difference between PPmax and PPmin, divided by the mean of the two values, and expressed as a percentage: ΔPP (%) = 100 × (PPmax – PPmin)/([PPmax + PPmin]/2). [1]

8. If the pulse pressure variation is 30%, what does this mean?

In this case, the high value of ΔPP (30%) suggests that the patient would be potentially responsive to fluid resuscitation. PPV is validated when the patient is mechanically ventilated with a constant tidal volume of at least 8 mls/kg and there are no significant arrythmias. False positive results may occur in the presence of right ventricular dysfunction. [2]

9. What do we mean by pulse contour analysis?

Arterial pulse contour analysis is a technique of measuring and monitoring stroke volume on a beat-to-beat basis from the arterial pulse pressure waveform. This has several advantages over existing technologies, as the majority of critically ill patients already have arterial pressure traces transduced making the technique virtually non-invasive and able to monitor changes in stroke volume and cardiac output on an almost continuous basis. [2]

10. What are the limitations with pulse contour or pressure analysis?

Physiologic or therapeutic changes in vessel diameter are assumed to reflect changes in Q. Put simply, PP methods measure the combined performance of the heart and the vessels thus limiting the application of PP methods for measurement of Q. This can be partially compensated for by intermittent calibration of the waveform to another Q measurement method and then monitoring the PP waveform. [2]

11. What is arterial pulse power analysis, and how does this improve the estimates of cardiac output?

This approach is non-morphology based, i.e. is not a pulse contour method. Power analysis is based on the assumption that the net power change in a heartbeat is the balance between the input of a mass (stroke volume) of blood minus the blood mass lost to the periphery during the beat. [2]

12. Tell me about the Fick principle. [2 for all]

Fick's principle states that:

> The total uptake of (or release of) a substance by the peripheral tissues is equal to the product of the blood flow to the peripheral tissues and the arterial–venous concentration difference (gradient) of the substance.

So, oxygen extraction (VO_2) is given by:

$$VO_2 = (Q \times C_a) - (Q \times C_v),$$

where C_a and C_v are the oxygen concentration of arterial and venous blood, respectively. C_a is measured from arterial blood and C_v is measured from mixed venous blood via a pulmonary artery catheter.

VO_2 is simply the difference between the inspired and expired oxygen concentrations and can be measured by respiratory gas analysis or estimated. The equation can be rearranged to calculate Q, which in this case is cardiac output (CO).

$$CO = \frac{VO_2}{C_a - C_v}$$

Equipment 9

You are reviewing a 75-year-old man, 4 weeks post mechanical aortic valve replacement. His case was complicated by an infected sternal wound, a hospital acquired pneumonia and, more recently, diarrhoea. He is struggling to wean from mechanical ventilation. The microbiologist has left a message to say that he has 'VRE positive' blood cultures.

1. What is VRE? What infections can it cause? How is it spread?

Vancomycin-resistant enterococci (VRE) are bacterial strains of the genus *Enterococcus*. Enterococci are part of normal gut flora. Some are naturally resistant to vancomycin, but most have acquired resistance by obtaining new DNA in the form of plasmids or transposons (transposable element of DNA). [1]

Individuals can be colonized with VRE in health or in illness, usually following contact with hospitals, especially contaminated surfaces or contaminated hands of healthcare workers. [1]

Common infections include catheter-related bloodstream infection (CRBSI), wound infection, urinary-tract infections and bacteraemia. [1]

2. How would you manage this situation?

The principles are source identification and control, appropriate antimicrobials and isolation.

Treat by identifying the source of bacteraemia – in this case it could be an infected line, an infected valve or from his sternal wound. [1]

Antimicrobial treatment may include the use of either linezolid, daptomycin, tigecycline or teicoplanin and will need close discussion with microbiology. [1]

Prevention is through isolation of infected patients, barrier nursing and strict hand hygiene with soap and water. [1]

3. What do you understand by the term CRBSI and CLASBI? What is the incidence of CRBSI in the UK?

Catheter-related bloodstream infection (CRBSI) is defined as a bacteraemia originating from an indwelling infected intravenous catheter. [1]

CRBSI can be defined as a bloodstream infection attributed to an intravascular catheter. This is usually determined by quantitative culture of the catheter tip or by differences in growth between catheter and peripheral blood-culture specimens and more thoroughly identifies the catheter as the source of the bloodstream infection.

Central line-associated bloodstream infection (CLABSI) is a primary bloodstream infection in a patient who had a central line within the 48-hour period before the development of the bloodstream infection. CLABSI is not supposed to be due to bloodstream infection at another site, but as occult infection is sometimes hard to find, CLABSI includes genuine CRBSI or bloodstream infection due to other causes. CLABSI is often used as a surveillance tool and probably over-estimates CRBSI. [1]

A recent published series reports CRBSI rates between 1 and 5 per 1,000 central-line days, although case mix and local microbiology are important factors. [1]

4. How would you identify a patient with CRBSI?

You might identify such a patient through clinical suspicion. There may be symptoms and signs of systemic sepsis; local infection at the site may or may not be apparent. However, there may be no other obvious cause for the sepsis apart from an indwelling catheter. [1]

Laboratory results can also identify a patient with CRBSI, through raised inflammatory markers, positive blood cultures or positive catheter tip cultures. Simultaneous quantitative paired cultures with a > 5:1 ratio of central venous catheter (CVC) versus peripheral cultures or non-quantitative cultures from a CVC that becomes positive at least 2 hours prior to a paired peripheral sample are additional strong evidence of a CRBSI. [2]

5. What are the principles of management?

The main principle is removal of any potentially infected lines. [1]

Empirical antibiotics may be used to cover likely pathogens (usually Gram-positive ones including methicillin-resistant *Staphylococcus aureus* (MRSA) but can include Gram-negative and fungal pathogens). [1]

6. How can you prevent CRBSI in the intensive care unit?

The use of central-line care bundles, regular surveillance and early removal of any unnecessary lines has been shown to reduce the incidence of CRBSI (matching Michigan study). [1]

Elements of a CVC bundle should include strict aseptic insertion techniques including appropriate hand hygiene, use of 2% chlorhexidine in alcohol for skin preparation, use of full barrier precautions during CVC insertion and avoidance of the femoral site where feasible. [2 for all]

It is important to ensure that lines are properly cared for and looked after once inserted and all interventions are done using aseptic techniques. [1]

7. What features of central lines help to reduce CRBSI?

Antimicrobial impregnated catheters have chlorhexidine or silver coatings. Catheters may also be impregnated with antibiotics, e.g. rifampicin. A Cochrane review in 2012 concluded that while antimicrobial catheters were associated with a reduction in colonization and CRBSI, this benefit was confined to patients in intensive care only and overall there was no difference in the overall incidence of sepsis and death across all studies. [2]

Equipment 10

1. **What are these two pieces of equipment?** [1 for each]
   What are the main differences between them? [2]

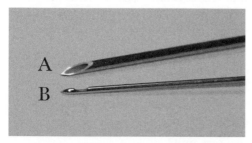

For the colour version, please refer to the plate section. In some formats this figure will only appear in black and white.

A. This is a 22G *Quincke*-type spinal needle with a short bevel cutting tip, which tends to cut the dural fibres.

B. This is a 25G *Whitacre* spinal needle with an atraumatic pencil point tip, which separates rather than cuts dural fibres.

The incidence of post dural puncture headache is significantly higher with a Quincke-type needle and is also related to the gauge, with a higher incidence associated with the use of a larger needle.

2. **When would you use this on the intensive care unit?** [2 for both]

A lumbar puncture in critical care is usually performed for diagnostic purposes. For example to assess cell counts and culture in the diagnosis of meningitis and encephalitis, the presence of xanthochromia in subarachnoid haemorrhage and raised cerebrospinal fluid (CSF) protein levels in Guillain–Barré syndrome.

A lumbar drain is occasionally indicated to manage CSF leaks post surgery or trauma. Examples include aortic surgery where the perfusion pressure of the spinal cord via the anterior spinal artery may be reduced temporarily. Reducing the CSF pressure improves perfusion.

3. **What other equipment do you need to perform a diagnostic lumbar puncture?** [1 for all]
   - Sterile pack – including drape, gown, gloves, mask and 0.5% chlorhexidine in 70% alcohol solution
   - Local anaesthesia
   - Manometry if indicated
   - CSF collection bottles – labelled 1 to 4

4. **What are the potential complications of lumbar puncture?** [3 for at least 4]
   - Post dural puncture headache
   - Spinal haematoma
   - Infection
   - Spinal cord ischaemia

- Nerve damage which may be temporary or less frequently permanent
- Complications associated with drug administration – including hypotension/autonomic blockade from the injection of local anaesthesia and wrong route of drug administration

5. At what level does the spinal cord end?

The spinal cord typically becomes the cauda equina at the level of lumbar vertebrae L_1 to L_2 (range T_{12}–L_3). [1]

6. What landmarks would you use for safe insertion of the needle to perform lumbar puncture?

Tuffier's line passes through L_3/L_4 and the iliac crests. This (or the space below) is the site typically chosen for needle insertion. [1]

7. How can we minimize the risk of injecting a potentially harmful solution into the CSF? [3 for all]

Use simple practical steps such as keeping drugs in different sized syringes, only drawing up what you need, checking drugs with a second person, discarding unnecessary or used drugs and carefully using and removing skin preparation solutions before opening the needle.

Specific non-Leur lock spinal needles are now available that will not allow standard syringes to be attached to the spinal needle.

8. Can you name some contraindications to a diagnostic lumbar puncture?

- Patient refusal [1]
- Local infection at site (systemic infection is a relative contraindication) [1]
- Coagulopathy/thrombocytopenia [1]
- Increased intracranial pressure [1]

9. You decide to measure CSF pressure using manometry. What is the normal range?

The normal range is 10 to 20 cmH$_2$O. [1]

Equipment 11

1. **Can you label the carbon dioxide waveform?** [2]

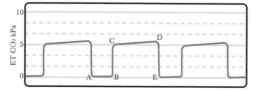

For the colour version, please refer to the plate section. In some formats this figure will only appear in black and white.

- AB – Baseline
- BC – Expiratory upstroke
- CD – Expiratory plateau
- D – End-tidal carbon dioxide value
- DE – Start of inspiration

2. **What is the underlying principle on which capnography works?**
Carbon dioxide (CO_2) absorbs infrared radiation. A beam of infrared light is passed across the gas sample to fall on a sensor. The presence of CO_2 in the gas leads to a reduction in the amount of light falling on the sensor, which changes the voltage in a circuit. The amount of infrared rays absorbed is proportional to the concentration of the infrared-absorbing substance (Beer Lambert law). [1]
Capnography measures the partial pressure of expired (and inspired) CO_2, which reflects the arterial concentration. [1]

3. **What different systems do we have to measure end-tidal carbon dioxide concentration?**
There are mainstream and side-stream systems. [1]
Mainstream systems are bulky on the catheter mount and may pull on the airway device or breathing circuit; side-stream systems need a pump and they sample gas from the circuit, leading to a delay in detection of CO_2. [1]

4. **How big is the difference between end-tidal and arterial $PaCO_2$? What affects it? Do you know some examples?**
In healthy individuals, the difference between arterial blood and expired gas CO_2 partial pressures is very small. In the presence of most forms of lung disease (anything that affects the ventilation/perfusion (V/Q) matching) and cyanotic congenital heart disease (or a big shunt) the difference between arterial blood and expired gas increases and can exceed 1 kPa. [2]

5. **What is 'collision broadening'?**
The presence of other gases in the gas mix changes the infrared absorption of CO_2 as the molecules collide with each other. The spectrum over which infrared light is absorbed

becomes 'broader' as a result. Nitrous oxide (N_2O) is a particular problem as it absorbs light of a very similar wavelength to CO_2. This is corrected for by either using very specific frequencies of infrared light (through filtering) or by measuring concentrations of other gases too and making mathematical corrections. [1]

6. Can you interpret these waveforms? [1 point each, max. 9]

1.

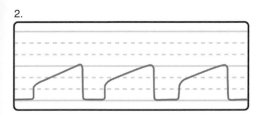

For the colour version, please refer to the plate section. In some formats this figure will only appear in black and white.

2.

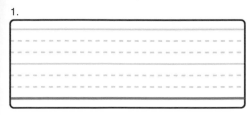

For the colour version, please refer to the plate section. In some formats this figure will only appear in black and white.

3.

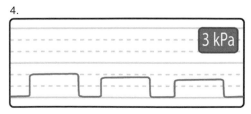

8 kPa

For the colour version, please refer to the plate section. In some formats this figure will only appear in black and white.

4.

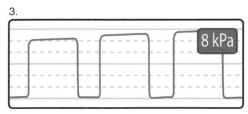

3 kPa

For the colour version, please refer to the plate section. In some formats this figure will only appear in black and white.

5.

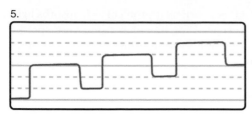

For the colour version, please refer to the plate section. In some formats this figure will only appear in black and white.

6.

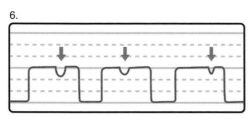

For the colour version, please refer to the plate section. In some formats this figure will only appear in black and white.

7.

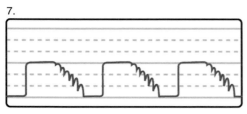

For the colour version, please refer to the plate section. In some formats this figure will only appear in black and white.

8.

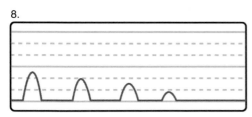

For the colour version, please refer to the plate section. In some formats this figure will only appear in black and white.

9.

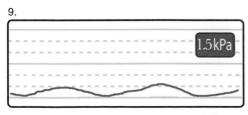

1.5 kPa

For the colour version, please refer to the plate section. In some formats this figure will only appear in black and white.

1. Flat line
   a. Disconnection
   b. Complete obstruction of lungs: e.g. very severe bronchospasm
   c. Complete obstruction/loss/displacement of airway: e.g. endotracheal tube obstruction
   d. Complete obstruction of capnograph sampling tubing
   e. Respiratory arrest (apnoea)
   f. Cardiac arrest: there is no circulation to bring CO_2 to the lungs
2. Upsloping
   a. Partial obstruction of lungs: e.g. bronchospasm, chronic obstructive pulmonary disease (COPD)
   b. Partial obstruction of airway: e.g. endotracheal tube secretions, kinking
3. Hypoventilation or increased CO_2 production
4. Hyperventilation
5. Re-breathing
6. Breathing against ventilator or during expiratory pauses
7. Vibrations from normal cardiac contractions
8. Oesophageal intubation
9. Capnography trace during cardiac arrest with cardiopulmonary resuscitation (CPR) ongoing

7. When should we use continuous waveform capnography in the intensive care unit?
[3 for all]

We should use continuous waveform capnography for all airway manipulations, including during tracheostomy.

We should use it for all transfers with artificial airway *in situ*.

We should use it for all invasively ventilated patients, including those ventilated with continuous positive airway pressure if via an artificial airway device.

Equipment 12

You are due to transfer a man with severe ARDS to radiology for a CT scan of his chest. He is on pressure controlled ventilation with a peak inspiratory pressure of 26 cmH$_2$O and a positive end expiratory pressure (PEEP) of 10 cmH$_2$O and minute ventilation of 8 L/min. His PaO$_2$ is 9.5 kPa, PaCO$_2$ 6.8 kPa, on 60% FiO$_2$.

1. How would you go about preparing this man for transfer?

First, you would prepare the patient:

- Familiarize yourself with the patient history and case notes; examine the patient and review any relevant investigations [1]
- Check airway, breathing, circulation [1]
- Establish team roles for transfer [1]
- Ensure the patient is adequately sedated and if necessary use muscle relaxants [1]
- Is the patient stable enough to disconnect and establish on a transport ventilator? [1]
- Establish on transport ventilator and ensure stability

You need to prepare the drugs:

- Check syringe pumps for ongoing infusions and carry reserve supplies of vaso-active drugs, sedative agents, muscle relaxants, etc. [1]
- Disconnect any unnecessary medications [1]

You need to prepare the equipment:

- Use a portable monitor, with all basic monitoring including capnography; check all equipment is appropriately charged and carry back-up power supply cables [1]
- Ensure adequate cylinder supplies of oxygen. [1]
- Make sure there is a standard resuscitation bag with all necessary equipment [1]
- Ensure familiarity with lay-out and equipment present in the CT suite
- Ensure all equipment is securely attached [1]

2. Calculate the oxygen requirements assuming a journey time to scan and back of 30 minutes. What cylinder size would you carry?

The oxygen requirement is calculated as follows:

$$\text{Oxygen requirement} = \text{minute volume (MV)} \times \text{FiO}_2 \times \text{time}.$$

Carry double the amount needed. [2]

The total volume required depends on whether your ventilator is able to entrain room air or not. Some basic ventilators will use exclusively oxygen. Oxygen flow is also sometimes used to drive the ventilator.

In this example (assuming air entrained by the ventilator):

$$\text{Volume of oxygen required for 30 minutes} = 8 \times 0.6 \times 30 = 144\,\text{L}.$$

Doubling this minimum volume is a reasonable precaution = 288 L.
An E size full cylinder will hold 680 L of oxygen. [1]
(C size is 170 L, D is 340 L, E is 680 L and F is 1,360 L)

3. **Clinical examination suggests that he is only ventilating the right lung and the endotracheal tube is at 28 cm at the teeth (previously at 24 cm). How would you manage this situation?**

Postpone the transfer. (A chest X-ray is arguably not needed immediately, balancing delays in not treating a likely problem with missing another pathology.)   [1]

Withdraw the endotracheal tube under optimal conditions (with pre-oxygenation, all airway equipment at hand, appropriate monitoring in place, sedation and muscle relaxants and direct visualization of the larynx). Reassess for improvement.   [1]

Carry out chest physiotherapy and use recruitment manoeuvres. Consider bronchoscopy. [1]

4. **His condition subsequently stabilized allowing transfer to CT. This has demonstrated a new left-sided pneumothorax. How would you manage this situation now?**

Consider needle decompression if there is a suspicion of a tension pneumothorax.   [1]

Insert a left-sided chest drain and connect to an underwater seal.   [1]

5. **Your consultant thinks that the pneumothorax must have occurred during the transfer. Apart from the above immediate clinical steps, what else would you do?**

You should fill in an incident form. The pneumothorax is new and likely occurred either immediately prior to or during transfer.   [1]

Equipment 13

A morbidly obese 60-year-old man is admitted to the intensive care unit with pneumonia, requiring invasive ventilation. He has a history of inflammatory arthritis for which he takes corticosteroids. He is lightly sedated to maintain tube tolerance. After 5 days on the ventilator, you are asked to see if he can be extubated.

1. What factors do you need to assess? [score 1 for each 2, max. 3 points]
- Has the acute condition resolved? What is his gas exchange like (P/F ratio)?
- Level of sedation/conscious level? Any suggestion that he will be agitated or non-compliant?
- Does he have an adequate spontaneous or triggered cough?
- Any concerns about a difficult airway?
- Left ventricular function (history, examination, echo)
- A spontaneous breathing trial (SBT) on minimal pressure support

2. Is it worth attempting a primary extubation? What do you need to consider?
[2 for all]

You can usually justify at least one attempt at primary extubation. This may require immediate, planned non-invasive pressure support or continuous positive airway pressure.

An inadequate conscious level, poor cough and repeatedly failed SBTs would lead away from a primary extubation.

3. What does the Trachman study tell us about these sorts of patients?

Early tracheostomy (within 4 days of critical care admission) was not associated with an improvement in 30-day mortality or other important secondary outcomes. A number of patients randomized to a 'late' tracheostomy were successfully extubated before 10 days. The ability of clinicians to predict which patients required extended ventilatory support was limited. [2]

4. What are the indications for tracheostomy? [4 for all]
The classic surgical indication is for relief of upper airway obstruction.

Around two thirds of tracheostomies are now performed in intensive care patients, the majority of which are to facilitate weaning from, or long-term, mechanical ventilation.

A tracheostomy is indicated where there is inability to 'protect' the airway (usually neurological).

It may also be indicated to facilitate 'airway toilet' (usually with invasive ventilation or pressure support) in patients who have inadequate spontaneous secretion clearance.

5. Are there any contraindications to percutaneous tracheostomy? [4 for all]
Most are the same as for open surgical procedures, although the percutaneous technique may not be as effective at stopping resulting bleeding, especially if the operator is not a surgeon.

Uncorrected coagulopathy, especially if dual antiplatelet therapies, can increase the bleeding risk.

Known neck masses, anterior vessels, difficult anatomy or a known head and neck cancer case are usual indications to at least discuss with a suitable surgeon.

Local infection, inability to palpate landmarks (or visualize with ultrasound), previous tracheostomy and a known difficult upper airway could all be considered as relative contraindications and at least require some planning as to who performs the procedure and where.

6. Does it matter if the procedure is performed percutaneously or surgically?

[2 for all]

The key concern is the maturation of the stoma. Most surgical tracheostomies can be safely changed at day 4 (some say day 2) as the stoma has been surgically created and stitched open.

There may also be stay sutures *in situ* to help open the stoma and elevate the trachea when changing tubes.

Percutaneous tracheostomies have been dilated and tissues will tend to 'spring' closed if the tube comes out within the first 7–10 days. After this, most literature suggests the tracheo-stomas are essentially the same.

7. Can you tell me what these different tubes are used for? [3 for all]

A. This is a sub-glottic suction cuffed tracheostomy tube. There is evidence that regular aspiration of secretions from the sub-glottic space can reduce ventilator-associated pneumonias (VAPs) as part of a bundle of care.

B. This is an adjustable-length (or flange) tube, 20 cm long (versus 12–14 cm for standard tubes). It is used in larger patients. (A National Confidential Enquiry into Patient Outcome and Death (NCEPOD) report suggested should be used in around 30% of intensive care admissions, based on body mass index).

C. These are fenestrated tubes. They can be used with fenestrated or non-fenestrated inner cannulae to direct airflow though the larynx. They are used mostly to facilitate speech.

A.

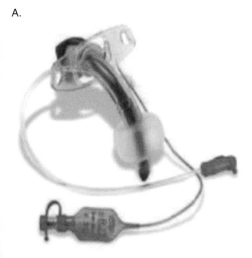

For the colour version, please refer to the plate section. In some formats this figure will only appear in black and white.

B.

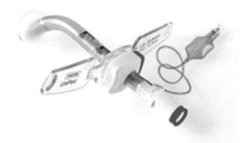

For the colour version, please refer to the plate section. In some formats this figure will only appear in black and white.

C.

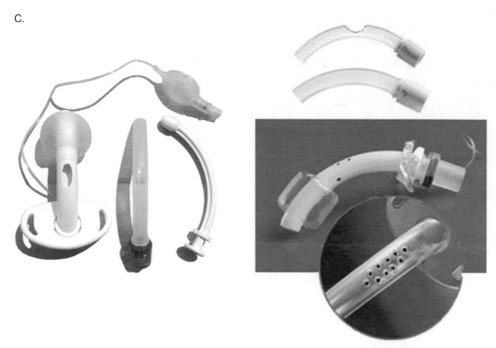

For the colour version, please refer to the plate section. In some formats this figure will only appear in black and white.

Images reproduced with permission of Health Education England e-Learning for Healthcare.

Equipment 14

A colleague inserts a central line into a critically ill patient on the intensive care unit and asks you to check the chest X-ray afterwards.

1. **Look at this chest X-ray and comment on your findings. What action would you take?**

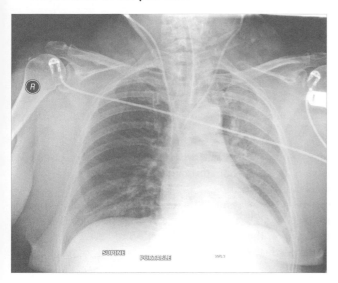

This is the chest X-ray of an intubated patient. There is ECG monitoring and there is volume loss and increased patchy opacification in the left lung, along with a small pleural effusion. There are three central lines *in situ*. There is a left internal jugular line with the tip laying in the left innominate vein, and two right internal jugular (RIJ) lines. The right-sided lines are of different calibres – one is presumably a vascular access catheter (vascath for haemodialysis) and one a standard multi-lumen catheter. Both tips lie well below the carina, with the vascath well into the right atrium. [2]

Two multi-lumen central lines are required sometimes when intravenous access is a problem, but this X-ray is more usual when a new line has been inserted and the position is being checked before removal of the old line (which may have vasopressor agents running). If the RIJ lines are not being removed, then they should both be pulled back into the superior vena cava (SVC) at the carina level. [1]

2. **Where would you want the tip of the catheter to be ideally?**

The tip of the central venous catheter (CVC) should be in a large central vein (SVC or inferior vena cava (IVC)), with its tip parallel to the long axis of the vein and outside the pericardial sac. Radiologically, this means that an internal jugular central-line tip should lie at or above the carina at the junction of the left and right innominate veins in the SVC, in a well-orientated chest film. It is important that the line tip is not against the wall of the SVC or RA, especially for left-sided lines. (Gibson & Bodenham, *BJA* 2013; 110(3): 333–346). [2]

3. What complications can a guidewire potentially cause when inserting a CVC.

[2 for ≥4 answers]

Guidewires have to be gently inserted and can be associated with the following problems:
- Cardiac arrhythmias
- Perforation of vessels or heart chambers
- Kinking
- Knotting
- Breakage of the tip
- Loss of the wire

4. What factors can contribute to misplacement of a CVC?
- Patient factors – difficult catheterization secondary to body habitus or previous failed insertions   [2]
- Unusual anatomy – for example a persistent left SVC or variations in the anatomy of the azygous vein; acquired factors could include stenosis or thrombosis of the vessel and extrinsic compression by a mass lesion
- Operator-related factors – including poor technique, inexperience and lack of familiarity with the use of ultrasound scanning   [2]

5. You have been called to assist a junior colleague who has inadvertently inserted a haemofilter line in the subclavian artery. What immediate action would you take?

Make sure that the patient is stable and not bleeding.   [1]

Do not remove the catheter as there is a large cannula situated in a vessel which cannot be directly compressed to control bleeding.   [1]

Obtain vascular and radiological advice on the best course of action to take.   [1]

Ensure blood is readily available if needed.   [1]

6. Are there any guidelines regarding ultrasound insertion of central lines?

NICE guidelines state that the use of two-dimensional imaging with ultrasound guidance should be considered in most clinical circumstances where CVC insertion is necessary either electively or in an emergency situation.   [1]

7. Can you describe to me what is happening at the labelled points of this normal CVP waveform trace?   [2 for all]

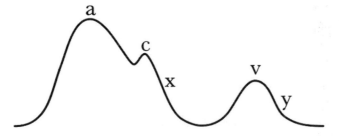

The a wave represents atrial contraction in late diastole.

The c wave occurs in ventricular systole and represents the bulging back of the tricuspid valve as the right ventricle (RV) contracts and pressures increase.

The x descent represents atrial relaxation – the tricuspid valve is still closed.

The v wave shows the rise in the atrial pressure as it fills prior to the tricuspid valve opening.

The y descent occurs as ventricular diastole commences and the tricuspid valve opens. The right atrium fills again until atrial systole occurs with the next a wave.

8. What is the difference between the normal waveform and these waveforms? Why?

[1 each]

A.

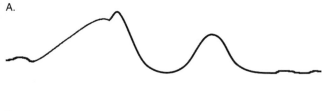

B.

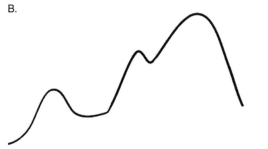

A. The loss of atrial contraction such as in atrial fibrillation results in a missing a wave. The rest of the waveform is dependent on ventricular activity and so remains visible.

B. In severe tricuspid regurgitation, the RV systolic backflow of blood out of the RV eradicates the normal x descent. The c wave becomes accentuated and fuses with the v wave, as both are the results of RV contraction. The v wave peak venous pressure is almost identical to the right ventricular peak systolic pressure in severe tricuspid regurgitation.

Equipment 15

A 65-year-old man has been admitted to critical care with acute kidney injury precipitated by a combination of diarrhoea, angiotensin-converting enzyme (ACE) inhibitors and non-steroidal anti-inflammatory drugs (NSAIDs). He is haemodynamically stable and still receiving ongoing fluid replacement but he requires haemofiltration.

1. **What do we mean by these terms: (a) ultrafiltration, (b) convection, (c) haemofiltration and (d) haemodiaylsis?** [4 for all]
   a. *Ultrafiltration* is the movement of water across a semipermeable membrane because of a hydrostatic pressure gradient.
   b. Ultrafiltration of large volumes of water across the semipermeable membrane creates a convective current that 'drags' additional solutes. This process of *convection* enhances the removal of small and mid-sized molecules.
   c. *Haemofiltration* is a process whereby ultrafiltration and convection are used to remove fluid and solutes from the blood.
   d. In *haemodiaylsis*, a counter current flow of dialysate is passed on the machine side of the membrane, which significantly enhances diffusion of solutes across the semipermeable membrane as the concentration gradients are higher.

2. **If we want to remove fluid from this patient, how do we do this?**
   Ultrafiltration leads to loss of fluid from the plasma, just like the normal renal function creates urine. If the haemofilter machine creates 1,000 mL per hour of ultrafiltrate, replacing this with less crystalloid per hour will lead to a net loss of fluid and volume. [1]

3. **What do we mean by the term 'pre-dilution'?**
   Replacement fluids can be returned either before (pre) or after (post) the semipermeable membrane filter. Pre-dilution therefore dilutes the blood in the fibres and reduces the tendency of blood to clot, reducing the need for anticoagulation and prolonging filter lifespan. Post-dilution effectively concentrates the blood in the filter, enhancing clearance. [2]

4. **What factors influence clearance of a substance from plasma?** [3 for all]
   - Membrane properties
     . Surface area of membrane
     . Hydraulic permeability
     . Pore size
     . Charge
   - Pressure gradients: hydrostatic, colloid, osmotic
   - Solute properties: size, charge, concentration

5. **Describe some methods used for anticoagulation whilst on haemofiltration and the mechanism of action associated with each method.**
   Heparin acts by binding to and greatly enhancing the activity of antithrombin III and from inhibition of a number of coagulation factors – particularly activated factor X. [1]
   Low-molecular-weight heparin (LMWH) therapy may be used – this also works through inhibition of activated factor Xa. [1]

Citrate prevents clotting by binding to ionized calcium in the blood. [1]

Calcium gluconate is infused post filter to prevent systemic anticoagulation and to avoid hypocalcaemia.

Prostacyclin may also be used, with its antiplatelet action. [1]

6. For which group of patients would you avoid using citrate anticoagulation?

Citrate anticoagulation should be avoided in cases of severe hepatic dysfunction. [1]

7. The haemofilter repeatedly clots. What are the common reasons for this? How would you manage them?

The clotting may be due to impaired vascular access. You need to ensure adequate flow and positioning. You might also consider swapping lumens. High intra-abdominal pressures and excessively negative intra-thoracic pressures can impede flow. [1]

If there is ineffective anticoagulation you need to correct this and/or consider additional pre-dilution. [1]

Ensure optimal haemofilter settings by setting the filtration fraction (ratio of ultrafiltrate : blood flow) at or below 25%. [1]

Consider whether or not the patient needs immediate restart of renal replacement. There might be a chance to assess renal recovery, unless indications for acute dialysis persist. [1]

8. What additional considerations would you pay attention to in a patient being haemofiltered?

You need also to consider drug dosing, correction of electrolytes, fluid balance and maintenance of normothermia. [1]

Equipment 16

This patient has been admitted with severe cardiogenic shock on intensive care. Electro-cardiography (ECG) and invasive arterial monitoring are in place.

1. What does the arterial waveform tell you about their treatment?

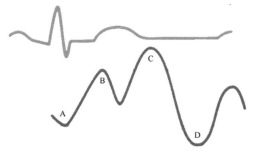

For the colour version, please refer to the plate section. In some formats this figure will only appear in black and white.

This patient has an intra-aortic balloon pump (IABP). [1]

2. How does it work?
'Counterpulsation' describes inflation of an intra-aortic balloon in diastole and deflation in early systole. This improves the balance of left-ventricular (LV) oxygen supply and demand by increasing coronary perfusion in diastole and reducing afterload in systole. [2]

3. Tell me what the points labelled A to D represent? [2 for all]
A. Unaugmented diastolic blood pressure at end-diastole
B. Unaugmented systolic blood pressure at end-systole
C. Diastolic augmentation of aortic pressure (balloon inflated)
D. Reduced end-diastolic pressure (balloon deflation)

3. Where is the balloon positioned?
The catheter is threaded up through the femoral artery and located in the descending thoracic aorta, distal to the subclavian artery and proximal to renal arteries. [1]

4. How is balloon inflation triggered and synchronized?
The balloon inflates with the onset of diastole (middle of the ECG T wave) and deflates at the onset of LV systole (peak of the R wave). [1]
Poor ECG quality, electrical interference, and cardiac arrhythmias can result in erratic balloon inflation. The balloon can be timed from the aortic pressure waveform. [1]
Inflation occurs after aortic valve closure, which corresponds to the dicrotic notch on the arterial waveform. Deflation occurs immediately before the opening of the aortic valve, just before the upstroke on the arterial waveform. [1]

5. **What are the indications for the use of an IABP?** [max. 2 marks for 3 or more answers]

- Post cardiac surgery, especially weaning from bypass
- Acute myocardial ischaemia or refractory unstable angina
- Cardiogenic shock, especially if myocardial ischaemia
- Refractory LV failure as a bridge to transplant

6. **Are there any absolute contraindications to its use?** [2 for all]
- Absolute
  - Severe aortic insufficiency
  - Aortic dissection
  - Existing aortic stents
- Relative
  - Abdominal aortic aneurysm
  - Severe peripheral vascular disease

7. **What complications can you see with its use?** [3 for all, 2 for most]
- Leg ischaemia
- Compartment syndrome
- Renal artery occlusion if balloon too distal
- Infection
- Dissection
- Perforation and haemorrhage
- Cerebral embolism
- Pseudo aneurysm

8. **What other mechanical therapies may be of benefit in cardiogenic shock?**
Left- and right-ventricular assist devices (surgical or percutaneous) may be of benefit. [1]
The use of extra corporeal membrane oxygenation (ECMO) may also be beneficial. [1]

9. **What are the types of ECMO do you know of?** [1 for classification, 1 for description]

The two most common types are veno-arterial (VA) and veno-venous (VV). Blood is drained from the venous system and oxygenated outside the body using an oxygenator similar to the circuit used in cardiopulmonary bypass. In VA ECMO, this blood is returned to the arterial system, offering a degree of circulatory support such as in the setting of refractory cardiogenic shock. In VV ECMO the blood is returned to the venous system.

Introduction

In the examination you will be led through various scenarios exploring ethical issues and testing your communication skills, some of which may involve an actor who has been given the relevant information and is playing the role of the patient or family of the patient. This section of the book gives examples of these scenarios where the role of the actor has been outlined. This role can be played by the person 'testing' you, or by a third person. Indicative responses are outlined below.

Ethics 1

You are asked to speak to the father of a young man 'Joe' admitted to the unit earlier in the day with a severe pneumonia and respiratory failure for which he was ventilated. He was inadvertently prescribed piperacillin plus tazobactam despite a history of anaphylaxis to penicillin. He has suffered a suspected severe anaphylactic reaction leading to acute haemodynamic compromise and a 2-minute pulseless electrical activity arrest from which he has been resuscitated. He currently remains intubated and ventilated and has regained cardiovascular stability.

Actor information

You are Joe's father and have been summoned urgently to the hospital as your son has had a 'reaction' to a medication. You are very anxious and want an update on his condition, having just arrived in hospital. You told a nurse and at least two doctors that your son had a penicillin allergy when he was admitted because you had a scare when he was a child – he became very unwell after previous exposure to penicillin.

Try and lead the candidate through the different domains below with your answers and questions.

1. *Father*: **How is Joe? I've just had a message to come urgently. Is everything alright?**
Introduce yourself. [2]
Go through the background including reasons for initial presentation and critical care admission. [2]
Discuss recent events including the administration of a penicillin antibiotic and its consequence. [2]
Describe the current situation – he remains ventilated and has regained cardiovascular stability. [2]

2. *Father*: **Why did this happen?/Everyone knew he was allergic/Didn't he have his wrist band on?**
You should apologize, admit an error has occurred and an incident form has been logged and a root cause analysis will be undertaken. You recognize the seriousness of the situation and should show a willingness to understand and explore what exactly went wrong. [2]
Tell him that you will order tests to confirm diagnosis (tryptase levels). [2]

3. *Father*: **Will he be ok? Will he have brain damage?**
Give an honest answer, that you don't know and we need to wait and see. But you can assure the father that this was a brief arrest and good-quality early cardiopulmonary resuscitation was given. [2]
Give the father the opportunity to ask any further questions. [2]
Be sympathetic to the father's concerns. [2]
Offer to update him again soon. [2]

Ethics 2

Please speak to daughter of a 70-year-old man who had a haemicolectomy for cancer (she didn't know it was for cancer) who is 4 days post-operation. He has now had a life-threatening pulmonary embolism and has been resuscitated from a pulseless electrical activity arrest after 10 minutes of cardiopulmonary resuscitation (CPR). He is currently intubated and ventilated and has regained haemodynamic stability. The patient was not on low-molecular-weight heparin (LMWH) despite having no contraindication to this and it seems this was omitted in error. His daughter is very anxious and upset.

Actor information

You are the daughter of the patient described above. You knew he needed a 'bowel operation' but didn't know exactly what this was for. You have not met the surgeons and just had limited information from the ward nursing staff who were always in a rush. Your dad was healthy and you are shocked that he has had a cardiac arrest as you considered his heart to be fine. You also had no idea he had cancer. You can't understand why he had an arrest and want a detailed explanation about the blood clot and why it may have formed. You also want to know how your dad's care will be affected by this set back and when he will wake up.

Try and lead the candidate through the different domains below with your answers and questions.

1. *Daughter*: Please tell me what is going on?

Introduce yourself.	[1]
Explore the current understanding of events.	[1]
Discuss recent events.	[1]
Explain that her father has had recent major abdominal surgery for cancer.	[1]
Tell her that he suffered a massive pulmonary embolism leading to cardiac arrest.	[1]

Assure her that the resuscitation was successful and he has regained cardiovascular stability.
Explain that the outlook is uncertain at this early stage. There was early and relatively short-duration CPR and a witnessed arrest but it is impossible to predict neurological injury at this stage. [1]

2. *Daughter*: Cancer – no one told me he had cancer!

Apologize for the lack of clear communication.	[1]
Offer an appointment with the primary surgical team to discuss things further.	[1]

3. *Daughter*: What caused this blood clot in his lungs?

Explain that there are multiple potential contributory factors including:

• The history of cancer	[1]
• His recent operation	[1]
• His immobility	[1]
• That he hadn't received LMWH prophylaxis	[1]

4. *Daughter*: Why he didn't receive prophylaxis?

Explain that is is unclear why; there was possibly an omission. [1]

Offer a sincere apology. [2]

Assure her that you will look into this as a serious untoward event and perform a root cause analysis. [1]

5. *Daughter*: I want answers!

Reiterate that you will fully investigate the matter as soon as possible and keep her fully informed of events. [1]

Explain that your current focus remains on getting her father through this event. [1]

Offer an opportunity for her to ask questions and arrange another time to speak to her again. [2]

Ethics 3

A patient presents for elective hysterectomy. After induction of anaesthesia she develops suspected malignant hyperthermia. She receives the appropriate treatment and has since significantly improved. She is now admitted to the intensive care unit and is currently ventilated and haemodynamically stable. She has biochemical evidence of early renal dysfunction. The operation was not performed.

Talk to her daughter and address her concerns.

Actor information

You are the daughter of this patient who was having 'routine' surgery. You want to know exactly what happened and why and want a lot of detail. You and your mum both need surgery under anaesthetic in the near future and you are really worried that this might happen to you or her again.

Try and lead the candidate through the different domains below with your answers and questions.

1. *Daughter*: **How's my mum? Can you please tell me what happened?**
You introduce yourself.   [1]
Give a clear understandable explanation of what happened.
Explain that malignant hyperthermia is caused by a reaction to certain anaesthetic drugs
used in theatre.   [1]
It results in muscle rigidity and breakdown, a high fever, high heart rate and a build-up of
acid levels in the blood and can cause injury to the kidneys.   [1]
Explain that the mother has received the right treatment and is currently sedated and
ventilated and stable.   [1]

2. *Daughter*: **What drugs caused the reaction? Did they give her penicillin? She had a wrist band that says she's allergic to it.**
Explain that malignant hyperthermia is a genetically inherited condition brought on by
exposure to inhalational anaesthetic drugs and a muscle relaxant 'suxamethonium'.   [2]
It is not caused by the inadvertent administration of penicillin.   [1]

3. *Daughter*: **Will she be all right? Is she likely to have any long-term problems?**
Explain that having received the correct treatment, her mother's condition has significantly improved. She does, however, remain ventilated and needs an ongoing period of close observation. She has evidence of early acute kidney injury which needs close monitoring. It is too early to predict the likelihood of long-term sequelae just yet.   [2]

4. *Daughter*: **Does this mean she can't have an anaesthetic again? She still needs a hysterectomy!**
Explain that she can have further operations in the future. However, precautions will have to be taken, including avoiding any potential triggering agents.   [2]

5. *Daughter*: **Do I have to be worried if I need an operation?**
Explain that it is an inherited condition and it is sensible to arrange for close family members to have appropriate diagnostic tests (genetic testing and/or muscle biopsy) to help.   [2]
Assure her that you will arrange for a referral to be made to a specialist unit that conducts these tests.   [1]

Additional questions for candidates

6. What are the initial signs that you would alert you to this being a problem?
- A history of exposure to triggering agents   [1]
- An unexplained rise in end-tidal CO_2, FiO_2 or tachycardia of no clear cause; masseter spasm after administration of suxamethonium may also be an early feature   [1]

7. How is this condition managed?
It is managed by:
- Discontinuing the offending agent and giving 100% oxygen   [1]
- Instituting cooling and the administration of dantrolene   [1]
- Treating complications including hyperkalaemia, arrhythmias, acute kidney injury, metabolic acidosis and disseminated intravascular coagulation   [1]

8. What causes acute kidney injury in this setting?
Acute kidney injury is largely due to rapid muscle breakdown and the subsequent release of myoglobin.   [1]

Ethics 4

Roger Smith is a 65-year-old man, now 4 days following out-of-hospital cardiac arrest and has fixed, dilated pupils. Your consultant has discussed potential withdrawal of treatment yesterday, and brainstem tests today confirm brain death. As the specialist nurse for organ donation (SNOD) is not available, please go in and discuss organ donation with his family. Mr Smith carried an organ donation card.

Actor information

You are Mr Smith's daughter or son. You were expecting him to wake up after his collapse and cardiac arrest but he hasn't done. The consultant spoke with another family member yesterday and said they were doing some tests to see if the brain was working but you don't understand what these involve or mean. You knew your Dad carried a donor card but you never talked about it. The candidate should ask you about donation. If they don't, please bring it up. Please specifically ask:

- You don't understand what brainstem death means – please explain it to me
- Is he dead then? His heart is beating!
- Will he ever wake up? In the films, people sometimes wake after a coma
- What happens now then?
- Can he be an organ donor? (if not asked by candidate)
- Will he be aware of anything? You don't want him to suffer

Try and lead the candidate through the different domains below with your answers and questions.

1. The family don't understand what brainstem death means – please explain.

Demonstrate empathy and sensitivity at all times through conversation. [2]

Explain that brainstem death means that there is no longer has any activity in the brainstem. This is the essential part of the brain to sustain life and is involved in automatic functions such as regulation of heart beat and blood pressure, breathing, consciousness, awareness and movement. Their father has permanently lost the potential for consciousness and the capacity to breathe. [2]

Use unambiguous phrases that do not imply some sort of continuing life. [1]

2. *Family*: Is he dead then? His heart is beating! [2 for both]

Explain that this may happen when a ventilator is keeping the person 'breathing' and the heart will beat on its own for a short period as oxygen is circulating through their blood.

A person is confirmed as being dead when their brainstem function is permanently lost. There's no way of reversing this and the heart will eventually stop beating, even if a ventilator continues to be used.

3. *Family*: Will he ever wake up? In the films, people sometimes wake after a coma.

Explain that, sadly, brainstem death is a specific, irreversible diagnosis. He will not wake up and will certainly die as a result, with or without continuation of supportive care for the other organs. [2]

4. *Family*: **What happens now then?**

Explain that their father has died. His body is being kept artificially alive and this is an un-
natural situation. Ventilatory support will be discontinued and because he will not
breathe, his heart will stop beating shortly afterwards. The timing of this is sensitive
and family members will need to be involved. It is not in the patient's interests to
prolong supportive care after the diagnosis of brainstem death.   [2]

You should raise the potential for organ donation.   [1]

5. *Family*: **Can he be an organ donor? (if not asked by candidate)**   [4 for all]

The first step is to establish that this is the wish of the patient. Clear indications include
donor cards or being on the organ donor register. Family members may know a
patient's wishes. The next step is to discuss suitability with the local or regional organ
donation team. You should explain that you will make contact with them and they will
assess the case. They are likely to want to talk to the relatives and take some details, ask
for consent forms to be signed and take some tests.

Explain that this process may take several hours and he may not ultimately be suitable for
organ donation. Supportive care will continue and sometime new therapies are started
in order to try and maintain the organs that will be preserved. Should the patient
deteriorate and suffer cardiac arrest whilst preparations and investigations are made,
then this means that they cannot be a brainstem dead (heart beating) organ donor.
Other types of donation (after cardiac death) are possible.

6. *Family*: **Will he be aware of anything? You don't want him to suffer.**

Explain that brainstem death means that the brain has stopped working. Some crude
reflexes may be present and the body may respond to surgery by a change in blood
pressure or heart rate, but none of the signals are processed by the brain as it has
irreversibly ceased to work. You can be 100% confident that he will not suffer.   [2]

Give the family an opportunity to ask questions.   [1]

Offer chaplaincy support if appropriate.   [1]

Ethics 5

Mrs Fergusson is an 80-year-old lady who has suffered an intracranial haemorrhage 3 weeks ago. She has some residual brainstem activity but has not regained any level of consciousness and extends to pain. Pupils are fixed and dilated. A CT brain scan shows hydrocephalus, old subarachnoid blood and bilateral cortical infarcts, but the neurosurgeons felt that there was no benefit from drainage in such a severe injury. Other organ systems are stable but she remains completely dependent on artificial ventilation as her spontaneous respiratory effort is minimal (but detectable). The consensus view is that her prognosis is extremely poor and that end-of-life discussions should continue to take place. Her children have asked to talk to you because they disagree with the previous discussions regarding palliation, and they wish care to continue.

Actor information

You are the son/daughter of Mrs Fergusson. You want the doctors to continue treating your mum and hopefully the candidates will explore why! Your main motivation is because you cannot accept that she won't get better, and that she needs more time. You want more tests and more opinions and you have heard of miraculous cases in America where people wake up after long comas. If challenged, you are not sure that your mum would wish to remain artificially kept alive in this state but feel that it is your duty to get the doctors to explore every option. Your mum wasn't very religious but you are and you believe that life should be preserved whatever the cost. If challenged, this is different to your mum's beliefs.

Try and lead the candidate through the different domains below with your answers and questions.

1. *Family member*: **I know she has had a bad stroke but I think she just needs more time to recover. Are there any more tests you can do to tell us when she will wake up?**
Demonstrate empathy and sensitivity at all times through the conversation. [2]
Allow the family to express their understanding of what is happening and build on their knowledge. [2]
Explain that further tests are unlikely to be helpful, but you may offer CT angiography, EEG, an MRI scan or evoked potentials. If offered, these should be with the caveat that they are unlikely to change outcome. [2]

2. *Family member*: **I've heard of cases in America and read stuff on the Internet about people waking up after comas – when will my mum wake up do you think?**
Offer a sensitive explanation of the poor outcome. [2]
Use unambiguous phrases that do not imply some sort of hope of recovery [2]

3. *Family member*: **Someone said she is in a 'vegetative state' – is she? What does that mean? What do you mean by coma?** [4 for all]
Explain that consciousness refers to both wakefulness and awareness. Wakefulness is the ability to open your eyes and have basic reflexes such as coughing, swallowing and sucking. Awareness is associated with more complex thoughts and actions, such as following

instructions, remembering, planning and communicating. There are several different states of impaired consciousness, depending on how these abilities are affected.

These include:

- *coma* – when there are no signs of wakefulness or awareness
- *vegetative state* – when a person is awake but showing no signs of awareness
- *minimally conscious state* – when there is clear but minimal evidence of awareness that comes and goes

A persistent vegetative state is a disorder of consciousness in which patients with severe brain damage are in a state of partial arousal rather than true awareness. After 4 weeks in a vegetative state (VS), the patient is classified as in a persistent (or 'continuing') vegetative state. This diagnosis is classified as a permanent vegetative state (PVS) some months after a non-traumatic brain injury (3 months in the USA, 6 months in the UK, or one year after traumatic injury).

4. *Family member*: **The last doctor I spoke with said that the medical teams will make all the decisions about my mum. That can't be right, can it? Doesn't the family get a say? Isn't there a law or something about this? What if we got one of those 'power of attorneys'?** (*Push the candidate to mention the Mental Capacity Act and to discuss lasting power of attorneys, etc. – she doesn't have a lasting power of attorney and can't get one now she is unwell.*)

Explain that Mrs Fergusson does not have capacity. Her treatment is therefore covered by the Mental Health and Capacity Act 2005 (in England and Wales) and the medical team act in her 'best interests'. The General Medical Council has clear guidance to determine the 'overall benefit' of treatment, balancing the burdens against the likely benefits. In this case, the burdens would seem excessive and palliative care would seem to be the way forward. The medical team are duty bound to ascertain what the patient (not the family) would wish in this situation, considering advanced directives, lasting power of attorney or any clear wishes that were made and recorded with the family, GP or close friends.   [2]

5. *Family member*: **So what happens then if you doctors want to 'switch her off' and we want to keep her alive?**

Explain that you are aware that this is clearly a difficult decision, but one that remains the medical team's ultimately.   [2]

The family should be offered support and the opportunity to meet again soon, perhaps with a second opinion or a number of other colleagues.   [2]

Comment

Usually the family can be brought on board by mediation, an internal second opinion or sometimes an external one. A doctor is under no obligation to offer a treatment that they do not think will benefit. Ultimately, a High Court order is required if there is a disagreement. The court will take into account the evidence for the patient's wishes and seek expert views as to the likely benefits and burdens of treatment as described above. Courts are almost certainly going to side with the medical teams if they have followed the appropriate steps but there are circumstances in which religious or personal circumstances may mean that the courts find in favour of preserving life.

The family should be offered support and the opportunity to meet again soon, perhaps with a second opinion or a number of other colleagues. Trust solicitors or the risk department should be notified. The best outcomes are usually achieved by working with the families and reaching consensus, but the external or judicial views are sometimes needed.

Ethics 6

A 31-year-old man with end-stage Duchenne's muscular dystrophy, fed by percutaneous endoscopic gastrostomy and dependant upon home ventilation via an un-cuffed tracheostomy, has now been readmitted to hospital with a severe pneumonia secondary to recurrent aspiration of secretions. This is his third admission in the last 6 weeks and he is now in established respiratory failure on the ward and has been referred to critical care.

This question is an exploration of the candidate's understanding of the ethical issues surrounding this case and is led by the examiner.

1. How would you approach this problem from an ethical perspective?

Ask yourself whether or not he has capacity? Take all reasonable steps to maximize his capacity to communicate. [2]

Explore issues around his current quality of life. [2]

Do not make assumptions on this based on your own views/prejudice.

If the patient lacks capacity, does he have an advanced directive, or is there a lasting power of attorney in place? [2]

If the patient lacks capacity, explore previously held wishes/preferences if there are any. [2]

Conduct a sensitive exploration of the benefits of treatment versus associated risks and burdens with the patient (if he has capacity) and/or carers. [2]

The main benefit of critical care admission here would be that of prolongation of life in what is a progressive terminal disease. [1]

The burdens and risks will likely include factors such as the need for unpleasant and potentially futile interventions, a prolonged stay in critical care with further complications such as ventilator-associated pneumonia and likely permanent need for a long-term cuffed tracheostomy tube with potential resultant loss of verbal communication. [2]

Treatment is at best life-prolonging and a thorough discussion around issues including wishes and expectations is essential.

The alternative option includes appropriate end-of-life palliative care. [2]

2. Your colleagues admit him to critical care, sedated and ventilated, but 2 weeks later has shown no signs of improvement despite aggressive therapy. The critical care team are contemplating a withdrawal of therapy, but the family are very resistant to this idea. Numerous detailed conversations have failed to progress the issue. How would you handle this situation?

Attempt to involve the patient as much as possible, seeking prior known views regarding end-of-life care or palliation. [1]

Seek advice from colleagues/multidisciplinary team. [1]

Offer to set up a case conference. [1]

Offer a second independent opinion – possibly from another unit/specialist centre/expert. [1]

Obtaining legal advice in seeking a court ruling may become a necessary eventuality.   [1]
Usually, life-sustaining care must continue whilst the courts consider the case.

A patient or a family cannot insist on a particular course of treatment if the treating medical team does not believe that this is in the patient's medical best interests. Patients can of course refuse interventions, assuming that they have the capacity to do so.

Ethics 7

You will be asked to perform a delirium assessment on a patient in a critical care unit. This station can be run using a single examiner, or two if possible.

1. What do you understand by the term 'delirium'? [1]

Delirium is an acute change in mental status with a fluctuating course characterized by inattention, an alteration in consciousness or disorganized thinking. It is a manifestation of brain dysfunction.

2. What categories of delirium are you aware of?

There are three main types: hyperactive, hypoactive and mixed. [1]

3. Who is at risk?

Most critical care patients are at risk of delirium, which is specifically associated with:

- Patient factors – elderly, underlying psychiatric disease such as dementia and depression, severity of illness, pain, immobility, sensory impairment, sleep disturbance [2 for most]
- Environmental factors – noise, lighting, lack of orientation to environment [1]
- Pharmaceutical factors – use of sedatives, especially opiates, benzodiazepines, anticholinergics and dopaminergic drugs [2]

4. How is it diagnosed?

It is diagnosed using a delirium screening tool, e.g. the confusion assessment method for the intensive care unit (CAM-ICU), which is most commonly used. [1]

There are other delirium screening tools available.

5. Demonstrate how you would perform the CAM-ICU?

1. Check if there is evidence of an acute change or fluctuation in mental state [1]
2. A patient is tested for inattention by seeing if they can squeeze a hand correctly on the letter A in a series of 10 letters (SAVE A HAART). [2]
3. Is there an altered level of consciousness as assessed by the Richmond Agitation Sedation Score (RASS) or Glasgow Coma Scale (GCS)? [1]
4. Check for disorganised thinking with four simple yes/no questions and a command. [2]

Features 1 + 2 and either 3 or 4 indicate a positive CAM-ICU diagnosis.

6. Why should we be concerned about delirium.

It is associated with increased morbidity (increased duration of mechanical ventilation and intensive care unit stay) and an increase in mortality. It is an independent predictor of cognitive impairment and post traumatic stress disorder. [1]

7. How do we try and reduce its occurrence?

Basically, we should look at the risk factors above and try to optimize or minimize these. For *non-pharmacological* causes: [3 for all, 2 for most]

- Optimize analgesia, mobility, sleep patterns and orientation
- Review sedation scores and sedation holds
- Treat associated organic disease, infection, hypoxia
- Review medications and avoid deliriogenic drugs
- Optimize nutrition and fluid balance
- Consider sensory impairment – ensure functional hearing and visual aids are available
- Reduce possible sleep disturbance – promote good sleep pattern; avoid noise and activities that cause disturbance during sleeping hours

For *pharmacological* causes:

- Consider treatment with haloperidol – but exert caution with prolonged QT syndrome and risk of torsades; there is no role for haloperidol as prophylaxis (HOPE-ICU trial; *Lancet Resp. Med.* 2013; 1(7): 515–523) [1]
- Other alternatives include olanzipine and quietiapine [1]

Ethics 8

A 70-year-old man, 'David Smith', post laparotomy for anastamotic leak, was recently discharged to a surgical ward following a 5-day stay in critical care. He has deteriorated acutely on the ward 2 days post discharge despite appropriate care, resulting in a brief cardiorespiratory arrest from which he has been successfully resuscitated. He is now sedated and ventilated and on moderate doses of vasopressors. His deterioration appears to be secondary to a hospital acquired pneumonia. Explain to daughter 'Jean' what has happened. She is upset because she feels her father shouldn't have gone to a surgical ward as he was 'still too ill'.

Actor information

You are David's daughter and have come into hospital to visit and find your dad has been transferred to the intensive care unit again. You are very upset about this as you didn't feel he was ready to be discharged to the ward and were shocked at the lack of monitoring and lack of nurses on the ward compared to the intensive care unit. You want your dad to stay in intensive care until he is ready to go home.

Try and lead the candidate through the different domains below with your answers and questions.

1. *Daughter*: **How's my dad?**
Introduce yourself. [2]
Explain the background and events leading to current situation. [2]
Provide information on current status of patient. Demonstrate empathy. [2]

2. *Daughter*: **Why was he discharged to the ward? I could see he wasn't strong enough to go.**
Explain that David has developed an unexpected complication in the form of a hospital acquired pneumonia. He was stable at the time of discharge and was reviewed by the medical team; they thought that discharge from critical care was appropriate. He was receiving all appropriate care including regular nursing and physiotherapy input on the ward. [2]
He was being kept under close observation on the ward but, unexpectedly, he rapidly deteriorated. [2]
Reassure her that a review of events, from the decision to discharge leading up to his acute deterioration, will take place and any issues/failings of care will be identified and looked into. [2]

3. *Daughter*: **Will he be ok?**
Explain that his condition is currently fairly stable although it is too early to predict how events will progress. He is receiving all appropriate care and being kept under close review. [2]

4. *Daughter*: **I want him to receive the rest of his care in intensive care and not to be discharged to a ward again.**
Show understanding of her concerns. [2]

Explain that it is currently too early to plan for this eventuality but reassure her that any planned discharge will only occur when his condition has significantly improved and when he is ready to be discharged. There will be regular multidisciplinary input into his care and any future decision to discharge will be based on this.   [2]

Assure her that the family will be kept fully informed at all times. Offer to update them again.   [2]

Ethics 9

A 75-year-old patient was admitted 8 days ago to critical care with Guillain–Barré syndrome. He is in respiratory failure and cannot cough adequately. He is profoundly weak. You and your colleagues have decided that he needs a tracheostomy. He is intubated, on continuous positive airway pressure mode ventilation and tolerating periods without sedation.

1. Firstly, what are the issues around obtaining consent for this procedure?
The first step is to establish if the patient has capacity, as defined under the Mental Capacity Act 2005, which came into force in 2007. Assessment of capacity in this situation will likely be challenging due to his profound weakness and inability to speak. [2]

2. How would you assess capacity in this patient? [4 for all]
Capacity requires:
- Understanding of relevant information
- Retaining that information
- Weighing up the information
- Being able to communicate their decision

Information must be given in appropriate manner and every reasonable effort made to facilitate communication. A patient may have capacity for one decision, but not another.

3. Your assessment shows that he does not have capacity? Do we need to obtain consent for this procedure? [2]
We don't necessarily need to obtain consent, although it is good practice to document this and record all communications with regard to this. If the person does not have capacity, we act in their perceived 'best interests'.

4. What other information would you like to gather before proceeding? [3]
We should find out their past and present wishes, especially any will or written advanced directive. Consider the patient's beliefs and values, which may be likely to influence a decision. Are there any current carers/next of kin?
Check if there was anyone nominated by the patient prior to losing capacity.
Find out if there is a lasting power of attorney (LPA) – the formal delegation of decisions to an individual: LPAs effectively can speak for the patient.
Look for any court appointed representation, for example an independent Mental Capacity Act advocate (IMCA).

5. What if a family member objects to a tracheostomy? Can they stop you performing the procedure?
If they provide evidence that the patient would not wish to have this specific treatment, especially if written or corroborated by other advocates for the patient, then possibly yes. They would not have LPA powers but it is unusual for a medical team to go against a family's wishes unless there are specific reasons to do so. [2]

6. How would you proceed in this situation?

A formal, independent assessment of capacity is required. Legal advice and probably a second independent medical opinion would be useful. The courts are likely to side with what the medical team agree that the 'best interests' of the patient are, especially if supported by independent expert advice. [2]

7. What if the patient has no family and friends and has no capacity? Who do we consult then?

We consult an IMCA appointed by the courts. [2]

8. What is an advanced directive? Should we always act on one?

This is a written view of the patient, documented and witnessed when they had capacity. If an advanced directive has been completed about serious (end-of-life) matters, this will usually be lodged with the GP too. This should be acted upon unless there is evidence that the patient may have changed their mind. It should be applicable to the current situation. [3]

Ethics 10

You are asked to check blood for an unconscious patient (Karen Path) in critical care needing a massive transfusion.

1. Describe how you would go about doing this using the images provided. (Assume that the expiry date of the blood is acceptable)

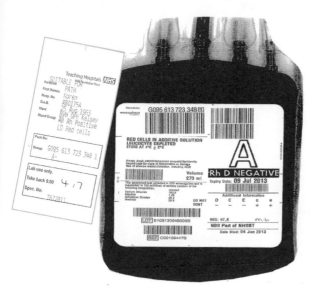

file in section 3

Pathology Directorate	Case No AB01754	**PATH**
BLOOD TRANSFUSION	NHS No	Karen
Compatibility Report	D.o.B. 25 Aug 1963	42 WHINNEY HEYS RD
Tel 01253 303746	Female	BLACKPOOL
		FY3 8NP

Specimen Number	Specimen Date	Specimen Date	Dereserve Date	Dereserve Time
T672811	02 Jul 2013	10:34	04 Jul 2013	09:00

RETURN THIS COPY TO THE BLOOD TRANSFUSION LABORATORY
THIS IS A LEGAL REQUIREMENT

Blood group   **AB Rh Positive**

Antibody screen   NEGATIVE

Lab Comments

GROUP A RH D NEGATIVE, NEG HT UNITS SELECTED
SELECTED UNIT(S) ARE KELL NEGATIVE

Product	Pack/Batch No	Group	Expires	Received by Date	Time	Sign	Commenced Date	Time	Sign
LD Red cells	G072 413 733 298 9	A-	09 Jul 2013						
LD Red cells	G095 613 723 348 1	A-	09 Jul 2013						

The persons administering the blood product must confirm that the patient
identification (Name, DOB, Hospital Number) on the wristband and on
the blood pack and the details on this report all agree.

Requested By	Requested From	Validated by	Date & Time Reported
Dr P.R. KELSEY	BVH OPH Kelsey	TB	02 Jul 2013
BVH OPH Kelsey			10:36

(Image reproduced with permission)

‖‖‖‖‖‖‖‖‖‖‖‖‖‖‖‖‖‖ Hosp No. AB01754

PATH
KAREN   15/01/1961   Sex : F
NHS No.

- Two trained members of staff are responsible for performing the patient identification and checking procedure   [1]
- The following details must be checked: [2]
  - Surname/first name
  - Date of birth
  - Gender
  - Patient ID number
- The above details must correspond with   [2]
  - Medical notes
  - Patient wrist band
  - Blood transfusion compatibility form
  - Compatibility label attached to blood pack
- The blood group and pack number on the unit of blood must be checked with that on the blood transfusion compatibility form and the pack compatibility label   [2]
- The blood bag tag must be returned to the blood bank as it is a Medicines and Healthcare products Regulatory Agency (MHRA) requirement that the fate of all bags of blood and blood products is known   [1]
- You should recognize the mistake on the provided images (blood bag and label differ)   [2]

2. What transfusion reactions are you aware of?   [max. 4]

- Acute haemolytic transfusion reactions – these occur when the recipient's serum contains antibodies directed against specific antigens on the donor red blood cells; for example ABO incompatibility and non-ABO incompatibility (Rhesus, Munro, Duffy antigens). These are often due to incorrect checking procedures
- Delayed haemolytic reactions – due to previously undetected antibodies and characterized by slow haemolysis and a positive Coombs test
- Febrile transfusion reactions – these occur when the recipient's serum contains antibodies directed against donor white cells
- Allergic reactions
- Transfusion-related acute lung injury (TRALI) – this occurs when donor plasma contains antibodies directed against recipient white cell antigens, for example human leukocyte antigens. It is more commonly seen with the administration of fresh frozen plasma, but can occur after red-cell transfusion.

3. Which blood group can you give to an A+ patient and why?

Patients with the blood group A+ have the A antigen on the surface of red cells and anti-B antibodies in plasma. This patient is also rhesus positive. Patients with this blood group can potentially receive blood from donors with the following blood groups: O–, O+, A– and A+.   [2]

4. **Your patient develops a new temperature of 38 °C during the transfusion. What steps would you take?**

Assess the patient for any other signs of a transfusion reaction such as the presence of pain (chest/abdomen/back), rigors, tachypnoea or respiratory distress, hypotension/hypertension, rash or urticaria. [2]

The recommended sequence of actions for mild reactions should include stopping the transfusion but leaving connected and rechecking the identity of the unit with the patient. If all is well, continue at reduced rate for 30 minutes and then resume at the prescribed rate. Continue close monitoring for signs of a transfusion reaction and give antipyretics. Contact the local laboratory for further instructions if in doubt. Significant reactions must be investigated further and the implicated unit returned to the laboratory. [2]

Ethics 11

These are the blood results of a 52-year-old patient with a history of long-standing alcohol addiction. He was initially admitted 5 days ago with seizures related to alcohol withdrawal and has now been referred to critical care with worsening respiratory failure and hypotension. He is drowsy, severely jaundiced and has a significant ascites. This is his first such presentation to hospital. His chest X-ray suggests pneumonia.

These are his blood results:

		Reference range
Sodium	128 mmol/L	136–145 mmol/L
Potassium	3.3 mmol/L	3.6–5.2 mmol/L
Urea	5.6 mmol/L	2.5–6.4 mmol/L
Creatinine	59 µmol/L	80–132 µmol/L
Phosphate	0.65 mmol/L	0.8–1.4 mmol/L
Corrected calcium	2.35 mmol/L	2.2–2.6 mmol/L
WCC	23.4×10^9/L	$4–11 \times 10^9$/L
Haemoglobin	9.4 g/dL	11.5–16.5 g/dL
Platelets	74×10^9/L	$150–400 \times 10^9$/L
Albumin	23 g/L	35–50 g/L
Total bilirubin	73 µmol/L	3–17 µmol/L
ALT	88 IU/L	30–65 IU/L
AST	77 IU/L	15–37 IU/L
Alkaline phosphatase	164 IU/L	50–136 IU/L
Glucose	4.0 mmol/L	4.0–5.9 mmol/L
INR	3.1	
APTT	37 seconds	28–38 seconds

1. What do you make of his results? What do you think may have caused the coagulopathy?
The low sodium, potassium and creatinine all suggest a chronic state and a dilutional hyponatraemia in the context of ascites is likely. The low albumin and raised INR suggest synthetic failure, especially of the vitamin K dependent clotting factors. The glucose is borderline low and should be monitored carefully. The liver function tests are all deranged

and an obstructive cause should be excluded. The low platelets and haemoglobin may represent chronic disease or consumption and the raised white cell count may imply active infection. [2]

2. What other investigations would you request?

- Septic screen [1]
- Arterial blood gas [1]
- Serum ammonia levels [1]
- Ascitic tap – send for M/C/S, differential cell count, lactate dehydrogenase, glucose and protein; if available, a positive leukocyte esterase reagent strip is suggestive of spontaneous bacterial peritonitis (SBP) [2]
- Chest X-ray
- Liver ultrasound scan [1]

3. The microbiology technician has left a message that there are 50 WCC/mm^3, the results of an ascitic tap. What does this suggest?

A peritoneal fluid neutrophil cell count of > 250 cells/mm^3 is usually diagnostic of SBP. In this case a low cell count and a low index of clinical suspicion, with an obvious alternative cause for sepsis, makes SBP unlikely. [2]

4. This is the result of a blood gas on 60% FiO$_2$. On 60% oxygen, pH: 7.28, PO$_2$: 8.9, PCO$_2$: 6.1, base excess –7 mEq/L, lactate 3.1 mmol/L. His chest X-ray is consistent with a severe hospital acquired pneumonia (HAP). How would you treat this patient?
[2 for all]

Admission to critical care is probably appropriate given that this is his first such presentation and because of the lack of a formal investigation. Early gastroenterology input should be sought.

Provide supplemental oxygen and titrate to O$_2$ sats and arterial blood gases. It seems very likely that this man will need invasive ventilation.

Provide multivitamins, lactulose and gastric protection.

Consider drainage of ascites if this is contributing to respiratory compromise and also albumin replacement.

5. Do you know of any scoring systems you could consider using in this case?

The Child's score is based on albumin, bilirubin, coagulopathy (INR), distension (ascites) and encephalopathy. This man is likely to be in the most severe (Child C) category. [1]

Another scoring system is the Model for End-stage Liver Disease (MELD) score, which is based on laboratory values including INR, bilirubin and creatinine levels as well as the need for dialysis. This is an alternative scoring system that was initially developed for identifying patients suitable for a transjugular intrahepatic portosystemic shunt (TIPS) procedure and subsequently used in patients being worked up for a potential liver transplant. It has also been shown to be of value in predicting prognosis in end-stage liver disease.

6. What strategies are of help in the management of refractory ascites? [3]

- Sodium restriction
- High-dose frusemide + spironolactone (an aldosterone antagonist)
- Non-selective beta blockers to treat portal hypertension
- TIPS procedure
- Liver transplantation in suitable cases

7. He is thought to have Child C liver disease. What are the chances of this man surviving?

The presence of Child C liver disease is associated with a 1-year expected survival of 45%. This patient also now has a severe hospital acquired pneumonia and respiratory failure, which is likely to further impact on outcome. [2]

8. Would you ventilate this man if necessary?

This man has advanced liver disease and a number of organ failures. The decision to invasively ventilate would be based on the likelihood of there being a reversible disease process from his associated pneumonia and if his physiological reserve is considered adequate. Given it is his first presentation you would think it reasonable that this be at least considered as a treatment option. [1]

9. Would you offer haemofiltration in the event of worsening renal function?

Worsening multi-organ failure and the need for renal replacement therapy (RRT) is likely to significantly impact on this man's survival and probability of a good outcome with a predicted mortality in this setting approaching 85–90%. RRT as a bridge to a potential transplant or to buy time for other therapies such as antibiotics to work could be justified. Faced with continued deterioration of multi-organ failure and decompensated alcoholic liver disease, some would reasonably consider haemofiltration to be not in the patient's best interests. Each case should be considered on an individual basis. [1]

Comment

This is an ethical question that you could justify either way. You often get the marks for the justification of your decision and not necessarily the answer. In the examination you are probably on safer ground to offer escalations of care rather than deny it, but this needs to be reasonable, discussed with the patient (and family, parent teams or colleagues) and balancing the burdens and potential benefits of aggressive, invasive interventions. If the examiners lead you into a situation where you want to escalate care but there is no capacity to do so, find a way, such as theatre recovery or transfers out of the hospital. It doesn't get any easier in the real world, unfortunately!

Ethics 12

This is the ECG of a 25-year-old lady (Jenny) who has been admitted to intensive care after having had a ventricular fibrillation cardiac arrest during a routine day-case tonsillectomy. She arrested shortly after induction of anaesthesia and was successfully resuscitated after 5 minutes of cardiopulmonary resuscitation (CPR). Her only significant past history is of depression for which she is on imipramine. She remains sedated and ventilated but cardiovascularly stable. There are plans to get an echocardiogram and probably wake her later today. You are not expecting neurological sequelae.

Jenny's mum (Margaret) is extremely worried. She has had an earlier update with the consultant intensivist but was not able to assimilate the information given. You are asked to provide her with a further update.

Actor information

You are the mother of the patient described above. You have had an explanation from another doctor but you can't understand why she had an arrest and want a detailed explanation. You are very anxious and ask lots of questions.

Try and lead the candidate through the different domains below with your answers and questions.

1. **What does the ECG reveal? (Offer the diagnosis if incorrect)**

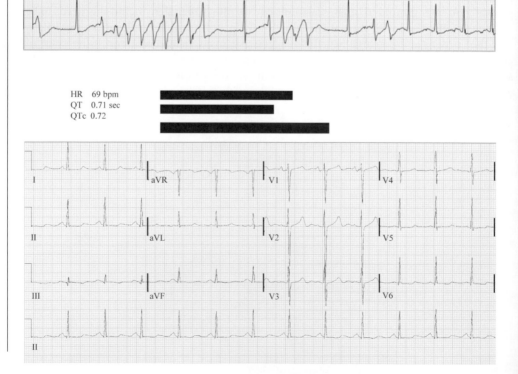

The rhythm strip is indicative of torsades de pointes. [1]

The ECG shows a prolonged corrected QT interval (QTc). [1]

The QTc estimates the QT interval at a heart rate of 60 beats per minute (Bazett's formula: QTc = QT/√HR).

QTc is prolonged if > 440 ms in men or > 460 ms in women.

QTc > 500 is associated with an increased risk of torsades de pointes.

2. *Mother*: Please can you tell me how Jenny is? I've been told she had an abnormal heart rhythm.

Introduce yourself. [2]

Ask for any prior understanding of events from earlier discussion. [2]

Explain the background events: [2]

- the unexpected cardiac arrest during elective day case procedure
- the early CPR
- the relatively short time to the return of spontaneous circulation (ROSC)
- that the diagnosis is unclear but may be related to an underlying heart rhythm disturbance

3. *Mother*: Did she have a reaction to the anaesthetic? Are you keeping something from me?

Explain that the event occurred soon after the start of anaesthesia. At this point in time, the exact cause is still unclear but thought not to be an allergic reaction. The ECG does show evidence of an underlying heart rhythm disturbance related to abnormalities in electrical conduction. Other possibilities are being considered however but seem less likely. [2]

4. *Mother*: She is a fit and healthy 25-year-old who does competitive sport including long-distance running and has never had any problems with her heart. Wouldn't something have been picked up previously?

Explain that patients with this condition (long QT syndrome) can remain asymptomatic or suffer from sudden collapse, seizures or life-threatening heart rhythm disturbances. The trigger for these events can include strenuous exercise and stress. The exact trigger for current events is unclear. [2]

5. *Mother*: What has caused this?

Explain that in general long QT syndrome is either genetically inherited or acquired. [2]

Acquired causes include low potassium or magnesium levels.

Certain medication can also trigger this. For example, certain antibiotics, antihistamines and antidepressants. Jenny is on an antidepressant and this may have contributed.

6. *Mother*: So what happens now?

Explain that you will keep her sedated and ventilated for the next 24 hours with the aim of stabilizing her condition and protecting her brain from any further injury. Assure the mother that you will ensure that ongoing cardiological input is provided. [2]

7. *Mother*: Could she have brain damage?

Explain that the early good CPR and a relatively short time to return of spontaneous circulation will hopefully significantly lower the chances of this. However, this is a potential issue and you will need time to assess. [2]

8. *Mother*: **How do you stop this happening again?**
Explain that you will take advice from cardiology. They are likely to suggest a need for further investigation and treatment with medication (beta blockers). Some patients may need an implantable cardiac defibrillator that is able to recognise an abnormal rhythm and correct it. [2]

Introduction

The questions in this section are presented such that a candidate could use the material either simply to read through, or could give this information to a colleague to facilitate low- or high-fidelity simulation scenarios.

The information is presented in the following sequence:

- **Overview**: This is a brief high-level overview of the scenario.
- **Key learning objectives/assessment criteria**: This states what the question is testing.
- **Background for candidates**: This section is typical of the information given to candidates to read prior to commencing a scenario. This could be read aloud or copied and offered to the candidate in order to prepare. Candidates should use this time to consider the likely key learning objectives and assessment criteria, along with the possible directions that the scenario may take.
- **Information for simulation facilitators**: This section details what equipment and set-up a typical simulation scenario based on this question would require. Due to significant differences between manikins and simulation environments, the guidelines are fairly broad, but will be able to be interpreted by those familiar with medical simulation.
- **Progress and mark scheme**: This describes what actions are expected from the candidate at each stage. It includes prompts and directions as to interventions or changes required by the facilitators in order to move the scenario forwards. Some of the detailed background knowledge asked and tested is listed in the next section due to space considerations in the table. Some common abbreviations used are defined as follows: BP, blood pressure; HR, heart rate (measured in beats per minute (bpm); RR, respiratory rate (breaths per minute (bpm); FiO_2: fraction of inspired oxygen; SpO_2: an estimate of arterial oxygen saturation; PaO_2 ($PaCO_2$): partial pressure of oxygen (carbon dioxide) in arterial blood; ECG; AVPU (scale), 'alert, voice, pain, unresponsive'; GCS, Glasgow Coma Scale.
- **Further information for examiners to facilitate discussion**: Information is presented here to help candidates and facilitators with the scenario. Further information that underpins elements of the scenario's key learning objectives that cannot fit into the mark scheme table is detailed.

251

Resuscitation 1

Overview

A 72-year-old male ventilated patient removes his endotracheal tube (ETT) and he requires urgent management. Demonstrate management of the difficult airway. Discuss risk factors for airway problems and preventative strategies.

Key learning objectives/assessment criteria

- Evaluate the need for reintubation
- Manage the difficult airway
- Describe risk factors for airway device displacement in intensive care
- Describe strategies to reduce risk of airway incidents in the intensive care unit
- Clinical governance: incident management/root cause analysis/morbidity and mortality/duty of candour

Background for candidates

You are called to a side room in intensive care because a male patient has removed his own ETT. He is a 72-year-old man with a background of morbid obesity (120 kg), obstructive sleep apnoea and type 2 diabetes. Three days ago he suffered an out-of-hospital cardiac arrest (ventricular fibrillation) due to myocardial infarction. On sedation hold today he became combative, so was resedated. He was left unsupervised by the nurse for a short period of time, then was discovered having removed his ETT. Vital signs are as follows: HR, 124 bpm, sinus rhythm; BP, 220/105 mmHg; RR, 40 bpm. He is cyanosed, agitated and is failing to obey commands.

Please demonstrate how you would manage this situation.

Information for simulation facilitators

Initial set-up

- Manikin laid on bed
- Two assistants to act as critical care nurses
- Arterial blood pressure, central venous catheter, ECG monitoring. Pulse oximeter on bed but removed from patient
- Intensive care unit ventilator/anaesthetic machine; capnography

You will need:

- Intubation equipment – basic: face-mask, Geudel airway, waters circuit, laryngoscope, ETT, laryngeal mask, bougie
- Intubation equipment – advanced: supraglottic airway device, cricothyroidotomy sets
- Suction apparatus
- Mock intubation drugs

Initial vital signs:
- HR: 124 bpm sinus
- BP: 210/105 mmHg
- RR: 40 bpm
- SpO_2 75% when pulse oximeter attached to patient

Progress and mark scheme

Initial assessment

Expect an ABCD approach from the candidate.

Action	Simulation action/response	Marking
Assess airway. Apply O_2. Call for help. Apply pulse oximeter.	Patent airway. SpO_2 75% rising to 80% with O_2	1
Assess breathing: • Rate • Breathing pattern • Chest examination	Vital signs as above. Laboured breathing pattern. Bibasal crackles.	1
Assess circulation	Vital signs as above. Clammy.	1
Assess disability: AVPU or GCS	Agitated/combative. Attempts to remove face-mask. Intravenous access at risk of being displaced	1
Check blood glucose	Blood glucose is 7.1 mmol/L	1
Elects to reintubate	SpO_2 continues to fall if chooses alternative plan. Proceed to PEA cardiac arrest once SpO_2 falls below 40%	1
Preparation for intubation: • Plans rapid sequence induction • Selects drugs (and doses) 　• Intubation drugs 　• Emergency drugs 　• Sedation +/− inotropes • Assembles equipment 　• Waters circuit 　• Face-mask(s) 　• Guedel/nasopharyngeal airway 　• heat moisture exchange filter (HMEF), catheter mount 　• Laryngoscope(s) 　• ETT(s) 　• Difficult intubation trolley • Monitoring 　• Confirms ECG, BP, pulse oximetry in place		1 1 1 1

(cont.)

Action	Simulation action/response	Marking
• Applies capnography		1
• Communication		1
• Assigns roles		
• Recognizes potential difficult airway		
• Verbalizes plan		
Intubation attempt • Pre-oxygenation • Cricoid pressure • Positioning of patient (head tilt, chin lift)	Failure to intubate: • Manikin set to 'difficult intubation' • No capnograph trace • SpO$_2$ 80%, falling to 70%	1
Manages failed intubation • Removes ETT • Calls for help (if not already done so) • No more than two further attempts at intubation. May consider bougie, laryngeal manipulation, reduction in cricoid force • Maintains oxygenation with Waters circuit, face-mask and Guedel *or* • Inserts supra-glottic airway device	SpO$_2$ increases to 90% Capnography trace present	3

Further information for examiners to facilitate discussion

- Explore further management of failed intubation or 'can't intubate, can't ventilate'
  - Use of additional equipment: videolaryngoscopes, fibreoptic scope, cricothyroidotomy techniques
- Describe risk factors for displaced airways in intensive care: [1]
  - Obesity
  - Delirium
  - Degree of sedation
  - Nursing staffing, care during nursing procedures
  - Time of day (more common out of hours)
- Describe preventative strategies: [1]
  - Use of capnography
  - Appropriate staffing levels (medical and nursing)
  - Identification of at risk patients
- Discuss clinical governance issues: [2]
  - Incident reporting: local systems, National Learning and Reporting System (UK)
  - Root cause analysis
  - Duty of candour

Resuscitation 2

Overview

A 3-year-old boy is submersed in bathtub at home. There was cardiac arrest at scene. Paramedics transfer him to the nearest emergency department, cardiopulmonary resuscitation (CPR) ongoing.

This station assesses knowledge and execution of paediatric life-support algorithms. Additionally, it tests specific knowledge of drowning and safeguarding processes.

Key learning objectives/assessment criteria

- Co-ordinate paediatric life support
- Look for hypothermia, demonstrate knowledge of management
- Management of patient following submersion
- Identify possibility of non-accidental injury (NAI) given suspicious circumstances. Knowledge of safeguarding
- Plan ongoing care

Background for candidates

You are the intensive care unit registrar on call in a district general hospital. A paediatric arrest call summons you to the emergency department, where a 3-year-old boy is awaited. You are the most senior doctor present. He arrives with paramedics performing CPR. You are told he was found in cardiac arrest in the bathroom, next to a bathtub (half full of water). His mother is following, after she has found someone to look after his three siblings.

Information for simulation facilitators

Initial set-up

- Paediatric manikin laid on bed
- Two assistants to act as paediatric arrest team
- Defibrillator (monitoring ECG). CPR in progress. Child ventilated via bag valve mask

You will need:

- White board or paper to detail drug doses, tube size, etc.
- ECG, pulse oximetry, non-invasive BP
- Intubation equipment for child – endotracheal tube (ETT), laryngoscope, capnography, etc.
- Rectal thermometer, blankets
- Intravenous/intraosseous access
- Intravenous fluids (warmed)

Initial vital signs:

- Pulseless electrical activity arrest

Progress and mark scheme
Initial resuscitation

Expect the candidate to follow advanced paediatric life-support algorithm.

Action	Simulation action/response	Marking
Planning • Calculate weight (approx. 14 kg), drug doses, tube size, energy dose • Request senior help, assign roles to team		2
Establish basic life support	No response	1
Follow 'non-shockable' arm of algorithm: • Intraosseous access and adrenaline (10 µg/kg = 140 µg) every 3–5 minutes • Secure airway, using ETT (5.0–5.5 cm internal diameter) or laryngeal mask (size 2). Attach capnography • Consider reversible causes	Return of spontaneous circulation (ROSC) after adrenaline and airway secured	3
Assess disability • AVPU • Pupils • Temperature (low-reading thermometer) • Glucose	AVPU is unresponsive ('U') Pupils are equal, size 2 Temperature is 34.6 °C Blood glucose is 4.5 mmol/L	1
Discuss management of temperature	Hypothermia common after submersion. Ensure patient dry, apply blankets/warming device. Any fluids should be warmed and gases humidified. Therapeutic hypothermia not beneficial in comatose children after cardiac arrest.	2
Assess exposure	Looks thin for age, slightly unkempt	1
Re-assessment	A: ETT or laryngeal mask airway B: PaO_2 16 kPa, FiO_2 0.8 C: HR, 124 bpm, BP 89/42 mmHg Capillary refill 4 seconds D: Unresponsive. Temperature and glucose unchanged Although the history is not suggestive in this case, full trauma evaluation, including cervical spine, is reasonable in submersion injuries.	1

(*cont.*)

Action	Simulation action/response	Marking
Action	Simulation action/response	Marking
What problems would you anticipate in patients following submersion injury	Respiratory failure due to aspiration of water causing atelectasis (loss of surfactant) and shunt Hypoxic brain injury Myocardial injury due to hypoxia	3
After ROSC, what investigations would you perform?	Arterial blood gases (ABG) Chest radiograph Full blood count and biochemistry (fresh water possibly absorbed via lungs, causing, for example, hyponatraemia and haemolysis)	2
How would you continue to stabilize the child?	A: Intubate with ETT if not already done so B: Ventilate according to ABG results. Apply positive end expiratory pressure (PEEP) (5–10 cmH$_2$O) C: Ensure vascular access. At least, give maintenance fluids (not hypotonic) Further fluid boluses and inotropes according to haemodynamic assessment D: Re-warm until > 36 °C Give sedation, e.g. morphine and midazolam Pass orogastric/nasogastric tube, as likely to have swallowed significant volume of water Needs discussion with paediatric intensive care unit and transfer once stabilized	2
Are there any other concerns you have in this case and if so what is the process you should follow?	Submersion in the home should raise concerns of non-accidental injury. If so, the child's siblings may be at risk. Appropriate personnel should be alerted, for example the on-call consultant paediatrician or designated doctor or named nurse for safeguarding.	2

Further developments

These will be post ROSC discussion.

Further information for examiners to facilitate discussion

Submersion encompasses drowning and near drowning (patient survives at least 24 hours after event) in children, most common in boys less than 5 years and between 15–19 years (associated with trauma, drug and alcohol ingestion). Prolonged submersion results in hypoxic brain injury. Ventilation/perfusion mismatch is seen with increased oxygen requirements. Aspiration of water washes out surfactant causing atelectasis. Multiple organ failure can ensue.

Hypothermia is commonly present. Traditionally, resuscitation attempts have been continued until patients have been warmed, based on anecdotal reports of miraculous survivals after submersion in icy water (< 5 °C). However, submersion in non-icy water does not confer neurological protection. When to discontinue resuscitation attempts is a difficult dilemma in the presence of hypothermia.

Submersion in the home raises the suspicion of child abuse. It is the duty of all healthcare staff to safeguard and promote the welfare of children and young people. In the UK, medical staff (who have some contact with children) are required to achieve competencies in safeguarding children and young people to level 2 at least. Competencies include describing different forms of child abuse, identifying signs of child abuse and recording and sharing concerns with appropriate individuals.

Resuscitation 3

Overview

A 2-year-old child presents with a traumatic subdural haemorrhage, probably due to non-accidental injury. This requires assessment, intubation, CT scanning and urgent transfer to a neurosciences centre.

This station will not assess actual intubation in the time allowed for the OSCE (but could be incorporated in longer scenarios if desired).

Key learning objectives/assessment criteria

- Perform a primary survey
- Select appropriate drugs and equipment for intubation
- Knowledge of maintenance sedation
- Interpretation of CT scan
- Recognize the possibility of non-accidental injury (NAI)

Background for candidates

You are the intensive care unit registrar on call in a district general hospital and have been asked to assess a 2-year-old child who is unresponsive and having generalized seizures. The child has intravenous access. On your arrival the child is having generalized seizures and has a large bruise over the right side head, although the mother is not sure how this happened. There is evidence of old bruising over the right arm and leg. Please demonstrate your management.

Information for simulation facilitators

Initial set-up

- Paediatric manikin laid on bed, fitting on if possible
- An assistant to help with intubation and act as emergency department nurse
- Intravenous access, ECG, pulse oximeter on (not recording if fitting), oxygen via face-mask
- Non-invasive BP cycling every minute

You will need:

- Intubation equipment for the child – bag valve mask, endotracheal tube (ETT), laryngoscope, etc.
- Mock intubation drugs
- White board or paper to detail drug doses and tubes
- Intravenous fluids
- Intravenous access
- CT scan

Initial vital signs:
- HR 131 bpm sinus
- BP 100/55 mmHg
- RR 30 bpm spontaneous
- SpO_2 96%

Progress and mark scheme

Initial assessment

Expect an A (with cervical spine) BCDE approach from the candidate

Action	Simulation action/response	Marking
Check/assess airway	Patent (oxygen already on)	1
Cervical spine control	In-line immobilization more appropriate for child, or collar	1
Assess breathing: inspection, palpation, percussion and auscultation	Vital signs as per info/monitor	1
Assess circulation	Vital signs as per info/monitor No signs of haemorrhage	1
Assess disability: AVPU or GCS Check pupils	Unresponsive Right pupil is 3 mm and reactive, left is 2mm and reactive	1 for both
Check blood glucose	Blood glucose is 5.9 mmol/L	1
Treat seizures	Stop fitting if suitable benzodiazepine given	1
Expose patient	Old bruises on limbs only	1
Paediatric-specific considerations	Ask for estimated weight (15 kg) Call for paediatrician	1
Reassessment and decision to intubate	Child remains unconscious (Drop SpO₂ if needs a prompt to intubate)	1
Preparation to intubate	Recognize need for all appropriate monitoring and equipment (prompt if necessary) • Capnography • Drugs with doses • ETT tubes • Skilled assistance	4

Further developments

Initiate a post-intubation discussion (practical intubation is not assessed in this mark scheme).

Action	Simulation action/response	Marking
The child has now been intubated. What drugs would you use for sedation?	Usually a combination of opiate and benzodiazepine as an infusion. For example morphine and midazolam.	1
What does the CT brain scan (see over page) demonstrate?	Large right subdural haematoma with midline shift	1
How would you treat the raised intracranial pressure (ICP)?	30 degrees head up
Normocapnia
Avoid hypotension
Normoglycaemia
Urgent neurosurgical review and transfer to trauma centre	1
The ambulance has just arrived to transfer. You notice that the right pupil is now significantly larger and no longer reactive. What would you do?	The child needs urgent transfer. In the interim could give either bolus of mannitol or hypertonic saline in an effort to reduce ICP.	1
Are there any other concerns you have in this case and if so how would you address these?	NAI should be considered given the severity of head injury and associated bruising over limbs.
Share concerns with a named professional for child protection or a consultant paediatrician.
Ensure accurate and thorough documentation.	1

Further information for examiners to facilitate discussion

Note the formula for estimating weight: (age +4) × 2 (usually underestimates).

Lorazepam dosing for infants and children: 0.05 to 0.1 mg/kg (maximum: 4 mg/dose) slow intravenously over 2 to 5 minutes (maximum rate: 2 mg/minute); may repeat every 10 to 15 minutes if needed.

Suggested drugs for intubation (15 kg):

- Thiopentone 3–5 mg/kg (45 mg)
- Suxamethonium 1–2 mg/kg (most use 1.5 mg/kg, making 25 mg approx.) or alternatively could you use rocoronium
- Fentanyl 1 µg/kg (15 µg)
- (Atropine 20 µg/kg) (300 µg)

Recommended drug dosage regimes include:

- Morphine for sedation dosed at 5–60 µg/kg/hr
- Midazolam for sedation dosed at 60–300 µg/kg/hr
- Mannitol as rescue for raised intra-cranial pressure dose at 0.25–1 g/kg

See www.crashcall.net for a comprehensive paediatric drug calculator.

Choose an appropriate sized paediatric ETT – 4.5 or 5.0 cm internal diameter.

The predicted size of an uncuffed tube is calculated as: (age/4) + 4.

The predicted size of a cuffed tube is calculated as: (age/4) + 3.5.

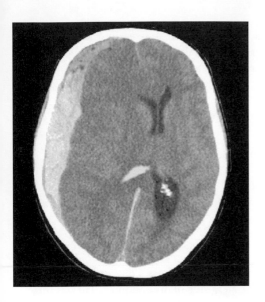

Resuscitation 4

Overview
A 68-year-old pedestrian involved in a road traffic accident arrives in your emergency department resus room. He was hit by a car and has sustained head and closed abdominal injuries. Balance the needs of cerebral perfusion versus permissive hypotension in the presence of haemorrhage.

Key learning objectives/assessment criteria
- Perform a primary survey
- Identify or exclude major life-threatening pathology
- Recognize acute head injury
- Recognize potential for acute abdominal injury
- Balance the competing priorities of cerebral perfusion versus relative hypotension for blunt abdominal trauma

Background for candidates
You are called to emergency department (ED) resus room to assess a 68-year-old pedestrian who was hit by a car at 40 miles per hour into the right side of his abdomen. He was thrown onto the bonnet and his head has shattered the windscreen. He was unconscious at the scene initially but was talking by the time paramedics arrived. He told them he had a past medical history of angina and a 'mini stroke' in the past but only takes aspirin and occasional glyceryl trinitrate (GTN) spray. He has oxygen, intravenous access and a hard collar *in situ*. The ED consultant is called away leaving you to lead the trauma call with an ED nurse. Please demonstrate what you would do.

Information for simulation facilitators
Initial set-up
- Manikin laid on bed with hard collar on if possible
- An assistant to help with intubation and act as ED nurse
- Intravenous access, ECG, pulse oximeter on, oxygen via face-mask
- Non-invasive BP cycling every minute
- No radial pulse *(if manikin allows this – might switch off with hypotension)*

You will need:
- Intubation equipment – bag valve mask, endotracheal tube (ETT), laryngoscope, etc.
- Mock intubation drugs
- Intravenous fluids
- Intravenous access

Initial vital signs:
- HR 125 bpm sinus
- BP 70/40 mmHg
- Temperature 36.1 °C
- RR 30 bpm spontaneous
- SpO$_2$ 85%

Progress and mark scheme
Initial assessment
Expect an A (with cervical spine) BCDE approach from candidate.

Action	Simulation action/response	Marking
Check/assess airway	Patent	1
Cervical spine control	In-line immobilization or collar	1
Assess breathing: inspection, palpation, percussion and auscultation	Vital signs as per info/monitor	1
Exclude the six causes of life-threatening thoracic conditions: • Airway obstruction • Tension pneumothorax • Massive haemothorax • Open pneumothorax • Flail chest segment • Cardiac tamponade	No significant chest signs. *Ask candidates if these aren't offered*	3 for all 2 for all if needs prompts 1 for some
Assess circulation with haemorrhage control	Vital signs as per info/monitor	1
Two large-bore intravenous cannulae Fluid challenge as low BP Look for occult blood loss: chest, abdomen, pelvis or from the long bones	*Ask candidate about blood loss if they move on. Can prompt by assistant saying 'abdomen looks distended'*	1 1 1
Assess disability: AVPU or GCS	*Moves all four limbs. Groaning, no words.*	1
Check blood glucose	Blood glucose is 7.1 mmol/L	1
Expose patient	Distended abdomen, bruising over hepatic area, obvious right-sided head injury, nil else	1
Investigations: • See X-ray vs. CT later • Bloods • Cross-match blood • FAST scan		1 for 3 or more

Further developments

Identify the goals of resuscitation.

Action	Simulation action/response	Marking
Targeted fluid boluses to resuscitate – see below	HR down to 100 bpm BP up to 110/70 mmHg Radial pulse back SpO$_2$ up to 90% with resuscitation	1
Triggers massive transfusion protocol Tranexamic acid		1 1
Reassessment ABCDE	Skip through this . . . Patient starts talking with a BP > 100 bpm	1
Disposal discussion: • CT scan or operating theatre? • Needs a surgeon • Likely head injury	Prompt for this Manikin deteriorates again during discussion	2

Further information for examiners to facilitate discussion

- What is going on?
  - Haemorrhage, probably intra-abdominal
  - Likely head injury
- Where should they go next?
  - Theatre versus CT – they are unstable; you could justify either
- What should we fix first – head or belly?
  - Stop haemorrhage
- What are your resuscitation end points in the bleeding polytrauma patient? (target BPs)
  - Permissive hypotension in the absence of traumatic brain injury (TBI): target systolic BP 80–90 mmHg or mean arterial pressure (MAP) $\geq$ 50 mmHg, if normal mentation and palpable peripheral pulses (prior to definitive haemorrhage control). The presence of central pulse is often quoted as a guide for penetrating torso injuries. (*Critical Care* 2010; 14: R52)
  - Hypotension (systolic BP < 90 mmHg) in the setting of a TBI is associated with worsening outcomes.

The primary objective of trauma care is to minimize or reverse shock thus saving life. Aggressive fluid resuscitation may be harmful in these patients because the resulting increased blood pressure and circulating volume may cause clot disruption, dilution of clotting factors and/or the reversal of the body's natural response to haemorrhage. The concept of hypotensive resuscitation has evolved where small aliquots of fluid are infused, with hypovolaemia and hypotension tolerated as a necessary evil until definitive haemorrhage control can be achieved.

Resuscitation 5

Overview

A 40-year-old lady with severe asthma is in the emergency department resuscitation unit. She needs intubating, and gets a pneumothorax.

Key learning objectives/assessment criteria

- Recognize indications to intubate
- Choice of drugs
- Complications of IPPV
- Recognition and decompression of a tension pneumothorax
- Discussion about subsequent IPPV

Background for candidates

Mary Smith is a 40-year-old teacher. She has unstable asthma and has been admitted to intensive care twice before but has never been ventilated. Her kids have had a cold for a week and she began to feel more wheezy than usual yesterday. She has a nebulizer at home, which didn't help today and so she took 40 mg of oral prednisolone and went to her GP. The GP sent her straight to the emergency department by ambulance as she couldn't speak at the surgery.

The emergency department specialist registrar calls you immediately to the (fully equipped) emergency department resuscitation area as she is struggling to say even words. She appears drowsy and pale. Basic monitoring has been attached, an intravenous cannula has been inserted and she has been given nebulized salbutamol via oxygen. An arterial line has been inserted. Please take over her care.

Information for simulation facilitators

Initial set-up

- Manikin sat up if possible but able to lay down for intubation
- An assistant to help with intubation.
- Intravenous access, ECG, pulse oximeter on, oxygen via face-mask
- Arterial line trace (speeds up deteriorations)

You will need:

- Intubation equipment – bag valve mask (BVM), endotracheal tube (ETT), laryngoscope, etc.
- Mock intubation drugs
- Equipment to decompress a pneumothorax – needle/syringe and chest drain, ideally
- Intravenous access

Initial vital signs:

- HR 130 bpm sinus
- BP 90/40 mmHg

- Temperature 38.5 °C
- RR 40 bpm spontaneous, with wheeze if possible
- SpO_2 87% on 15 litres non-rebreather mask

Progress and mark scheme

Initial assessment

Expect an ABCDE approach from the candidate.

Action	Simulation action/response	Marking
Check/assess airway	Patent	1
Assess breathing	Vital signs as per info/monitor	1
Assess circulation	Vital signs as per info/monitor	
Immediate treatment	Magnesium Continuous nebulized bronchodilator Aminophylline/intravenous salbutamol	max. 2
Ask for blood gas	*Offer blood gas if not asked for quickly*	1
Interpret blood gas	Give to candidate	1
Decide to intubate		1
Justify choice of induction agent	Ask them why they would choose. Ketamine probably best, but if they can justify another, ok	1
Justify choice of muscle relaxant	Would you use Suxamethonium? • Pro – classic rapid sequence intubation (RSI) • Con – bronchospasm risks Not atracurium, but rocuronium probably reasonable if they can describe potential problems and means of reversal	1

Perform safe RSI

Action	Simulation action/response	Marking
Cricoid from assistant		1
Pre-oxygenate	Drop SpO_2 to 80%	1
Administer drugs	Hypotensive 60/35 mmHg Apnoea Desaturate to 70% Allow easy intubation	
	If candidate can't intubate, get assistant to take over and pass ETT. Don't let the intubation practical skill delay the scenario	
	Capnography trace *on*	

(cont.)

Action	Simulation action/response	Marking
Administer vasopressor/ adrenaline		1
Ventilate with BVM	Set right-sided tension pneumothorax	1
	Assistant takes over ventilation with BVM and ventilates aggressively	

Further developments

Manage tension pneumothorax: SpO_2 doesn't come up post intubation.

Action	Simulation action/response	Marking
SpO_2 increases to 80% post ETT and BP improves slightly, then both drop again	*SpO_2 70–80 to 70% again* *BP 60 – 80 – 70 systolic* *Whilst candidate checks patient hopefully!*	
Check patient post ETT. 'Why are they hypoxic?' • Oesophageal intubation? • Endobronchial ETT? • Pneumothorax	Ensure right-side breath sounds absent. Ensure capnography Candidate may pull back ETT slightly – no difference Resonant percussion on right side if candidate asks	3 for considering all differentials
Confirm clinical signs of tension pneumothorax (ask them) • Absent breath sounds • Resonant PN • Trachea deviates		2 for all
Needle decompression	Release tension pneumothorax	1
Arrange definitive chest drain and chest X-ray		1

Additional information

Arterial blood gases for candidates:

pH	7.28
$PaCO_2$	6.5 kPa
PaO_2	8.8 kPa
Base excess	−9.5
Bicarbonate	16.2 mmol/L
Glucose	9.1 mmol/L
Haematocrit	0.41
Haemoglobin	13.9 g/dL

Resuscitation 6

Overview

A 35-year-old, 34-weeks pregnant lady is admitted to the emergency department following a collapse at home. She is acutely short of breath and rapidly develops a ventricular fibrillation (VF) arrest. The focus of the scenario is initial assessment and recognition and management of the arrest. Special circumstances include manual uterine displacement and early intubation. The likely diagnosis of pulmonary embolism is not addressed as the treatment is controversial in this setting.

Key learning objectives/assessment criteria

- Rapidly assess the patient
- Recognition of shock
- Initial assessment and management of acute shock and respiratory failure in pregnancy
- Perform a safe defibrillation
- Recognize need for early delivery and early obstetric input

Background for candidates

A 35-year-old, 34-weeks pregnant lady is admitted to the emergency department following a collapse at home. She is acutely short of breath. You are asked to assess her.

Information for simulation facilitators
Initial set-up

- Manikin laid on bed with a gravid uterus. Flat on back
- An assistant who is the emergency department (ED) nurse
- Ideally another assistant who is another ED nurse, but this role could be fulfilled by the examiner asking questions
- Intravenous access, ECG not on, but available
- Defibrillation pads
- No SpO$_2$ trace/reading (if manikin allows this – might switch off with hypotension)

You will need:
- Training defibrillator
- Intravenous fluids
- Intravenous access
- 'Bump'
- Intubation equipment
- Two assistants for the cardiopulmonary resuscitation (CPR)/airway management

Initial vital signs:
- BP 70/40 mmHg
- Heart rate 130 bpm regular
- Capillary refill 5 seconds
- Peripheral SpO$_2$ un-recordable (or 50% if this setting not possible)

Progress and mark scheme

Expect an ABCDE approach from the candidate.

Action	Simulation action/response	Marking
Check/assess airway	Patent airway, groaning	1
Apply high-flow oxygen via suitable face-mask		1
Assess breathing: • Inspection, palpation, percussion and auscultation • Check O$_2$ saturation	Air entry symmetrical with no added sounds O$_2$ saturations from pulse oximeter not recording	1 for assessment plus oximetry
Assess circulation • HR, BP, capillary refill • Attach defibrillator or ECG	*BP 70/40 mmHg* *Heart rate 130 regular,* *capillary refill 5 seconds*	1
Large-bore intravenous access Blood for full blood count, urea and electrolytes, cross-match Fluid challenge as low BP Arterial blood gas		2 for all
Ensure manual displacement of uterus		1
Assess disability: AVPU or GCS Check blood glucose	Groaning Blood glucose is 5.3 mmol/L	1 for both
Expose patient	Nil to find, other than a gravid uterus	1

Further developments

The patient at this time becomes unresponsive. Nurse assistant may prompt by asking the patient 'are you alright?' Manikin goes into VF. This may be detected if the candidate has already attached ECG or defibrillation pads, but will require reassessment.

Action	Simulation action/response	Marking
Re-assess ABC	Patient unresponsive. Not breathing and no pulse felt.	1
Call for help including obstetric team		1
Start CPR promptly		1
Demonstrate adequacy of chest compressions 30:2 ratio	*Candidate should be able to take an overview of the arrest – two helpers to manage airway and CPR*	1
Attach defibrillator pads	VF rhythm	1
Recognize VF arrest		1
Perform safe defibrillation including recommencing CPR immediately		1
Recognition for the need to intubate early (gas exchange and aspiration risk)	*Do not expect intubation – state that assistant can prepare*	1
Assess for 4 'H's and 4 'T's	*Assistant may prompt 'why do you think she might have arrested?'* Hypotension, hypoxia, hyper/hypo kalaemia/thermia Toxins, thrombo-embolism, tamponade, tension pneumothorax	2 for all
Recognize need for emergency caesarean section		1

The scenario tests cardiac arrest management and does not end. In practice scenarios, everyone might feel better if sinus rythm is restored and the baby is planned for delivery!

Resuscitation 7

Overview

A 66-year-old man has had triple vessel 'on-pump' coronary artery bypass grafting (CABG) performed earlier today and remains sedated on the cardiac intensive care unit. He is cold and mildly coagulopathic but has also developed an anastomotic leak leading to cardiac tamponade. This requires rapid planning for chest re-opening.

Key learning objectives/assessment criteria

- Rapidly assess the patient
- Identify or exclude common post CABG causes for hypotension
- Recognize bleeding
- Knowledge of 'medical' versus 'surgical' bleeding
- Rapid preparation for re-opening the chest
- Simultaneous assessment and management

Background for candidates

A 66-year-old man has had triple vessel 'on-pump' CABG performed earlier today and he has returned sedated and ventilated from the operating theatre to cardiac intensive care. The nurse looking after him asks you to review him as his blood pressure has been steadily dropping in the 20 minutes since the theatre anaesthetist handed him over. The procedure was fairly straightforward and the patient had been well until presenting with unstable angina 3 weeks ago.

Information for simulation facilitators

Initial set-up

- Manikin laid on bed and set up as an intensive care patient – intubated orally
- Manikin still ventilated (set to spontaneous breathing with capnograph) or ventilate if you have the facility to do so
- An assistant who is the intensive care nurse
- Ideally another assistant who is the surgeon, but this role could be fulfilled by the examiner asking questions
- Intravenous access, ECG, pulse oximeter on, arterial and central venous pressure (CVP) lines
- No radial pulse (if manikin allows this – you might switch off with hypotension)

You will need:
- Mock induction and vasopressor drugs
- Intravenous fluids
- Intravenous access
- Dressing over centre of chest if possible (sternotomy)
- Bilateral chest drains *in situ*

Initial vital signs:

- HR 125 bpm sinus
- Invasive arterial BP 75/45 mmHg
- CVP 25 mmHg
- Temperature 36.3 °C
- RR 16 bpm 'ventilated'
- SpO$_2$ 96%
- Heart sounds may be set to 'tamponade' or 'muffled' but these are difficult to hear usually in clinical practice and simulations, therefore not marked in this scenario

Progress and mark scheme

Initial assessment

Expect an ABCDE approach from the candidate.

Action	Simulation action/response	Marking
Assess airway	Patent – endotracheal tube (ETT) *in situ*, CO$_2$	1
Assess breathing: inspection, palpation, percussion and auscultation	Vital signs as per info/monitor Chest rises equally	1
Exclude tension pneumothorax and massive haemothorax: • Drains not kinked • Good air entry bilaterally • Normal airway pressures • Minimal blood in drains • Haemoglobin 'ok'	No significant chest signs No blood in drain Haemoglobin 12.1 g/dL on arterial blood gas (ABG)	1 1
Assess circulation	Vital signs as per info/monitor	
Note tachycardia/hypotension Note raised CVP Fluid challenge Vasoconstrictor bolus would be reasonable Echocardiogram (transthoracic realistically but transoesophageal would be acceptable) – may be requested earlier or later	*Nurse prompts candidate to comment on the CVP if not offered spontaneously* *Patient is cold peripherally (i.e. not vasodilated or 'septic')*	1 1 1 1 1
Assess disability/exposure • Appropriately sedated • Expose patient	*Drop BP to 55/35 mmHg, HR 135 bpm sinus rhythm* No obvious other problems	1
Call for help – specifically a cardio-thoracic surgeon		1

Further developments: diagnosis and assessment of bleeding

This section is led by questioning from the nursing assistant following completion of the initial assessment above:

- 'What do you think is going on?'
- 'Why do you think he is bleeding?'
- 'What should we do?'

Action	Simulation action/response	Marking
'Medical' vs. 'surgical' bleeding		
• Check temperature	Temperature 36.3 °C	1
• Check activated clotting time (ACT)	ACT = 160 seconds (normal 100–120)	1
• Check platelet count	Full blood count, ABG and	1
• Check ABG for acidosis	TEG can be ordered	
• Request thromboelastograph (TEG)		
• Echocardiogram (see above)	Echocardiography machine will be located	
• Surgical review (see above)	(move on)	
Correction of residual heparin effect (raised ACT)	Don't expect a protamine dose calculation (can state a perfusionist can help with that)	1
• Give protamine *slow* bolus	(Idiopathic 'protamine reaction' includes	
• Protamine 25–50 mg intravenously	mild pulmonary hypertension, hypoxia, and systemic hypotension)	

Further developments: preparation for re-opening (sternotomy)

A colleague performs an echocardiogram that clearly shows a tamponade. The surgeon wants to open the patient's chest immediately on the intensive care unit.

Action	Simulation action/response	Marking
The surgeon arrives (or could be on the phone) and asks you if you think this could be a tamponade?		
Yes. Mild coagulopathy but high filling pressures, low cardiac output, narrow pulse pressure and recent surgery make tamponade likely.		1
The nurse asks 'What do you want me to do about the blood pressure?'		

(*cont.*)

Action	Simulation action/response	Marking
Principles are high filling pressures, a relative tachycardia and a degree of vasoconstriction: • Fluid bolus • Vasocontrictor bolus or infusion	BP still 55/35 mmHg BP rises to 85/45 mmHg in response if treated appropriately	1 for both
Nurse asks 'Do we need to prepare anything else?'		
Need blood immediately available		1
Rapid infusion device or large-bore cannula/ CVC lumen		1
Opiates		1

Stop the scenario prior to sternotomy. You can continue to make 'preparations' for sternotomy and the candidate may be prompted to discuss clinical signs of tamponade if time allows.

Resuscitation 8

Overview

A 4-year-old boy (Jack) has been brought to the emergency department by his mum. He is poorly responsive, pale and floppy. A relevant history is required from his mum and then prompt assessment and resuscitation. The child has meningitis and needs rapid antibiotics and then plans for intubation when he does not respond to initial resuscitation attempts. The scenario is testing planning and management, not actual intubation (although, in a longer practice scenario, this is possible).

Key learning objectives/assessment criteria

- Rapidly assess the patient
- Knowledge of paediatric assessment
- Knowledge of fluid bolus doses
- Knowledge of induction drugs and intubation equipment in a child

Background for candidates

A 4-year-old boy (Jack) has been brought to the emergency department by his mum. His mum is concerned that Jack has had a temperature since yesterday, but this morning when she went to wake him she noticed that he was poorly responsive, pale and floppy. Please ask his mum any relevant questions and then assess Jack.

Information for simulation facilitators

Initial set-up

- Paediatric manikin laid on bed; rash on abdomen if possible (initially covered)
- An assistant playing the role of mum (or dad)
- An assistant who is the emergency department nurse
- In response to questions about Jack initially:
  . Past medical history: nil
  . No previous attendances or hospital admissions
  . Family history: nil of note, no sibling
  . Drug history: no regular meds, immunizations up to date
  . Allergies: nil

You will need:

- Mock induction and vasopressor drugs
- Intravenous fluids
- Intravenous access
- Airway equipment including capnography and a range of endotracheal tubes (ETTs)

Initial vital signs:
- HR 160 bpm regular
- BP 70/40 mmHg
- Temperature 38.5 °C
- RR 45 bpm spontaneous
- SpO$_2$ 94% room air

Progress and mark scheme
Initial assessment
Expect an ABCDE approach from the candidate.

Action	Simulation action/response	Marking
Assess airway	Patent	1
Assess breathing • Inspection, palpation, percussion and auscultation • High-flow oxygen	Normal chest signs	1 1
Assess circulation	Vital signs as per info/monitor	1
Assess disability Check glucose	P on AVPU, PEARL No localizing signs Blood glucose is 6.8 mmol/L	1 1
Expose patient	Widespread petechial non-blanching rash	1
Call for help – specifically a paediatrician		1
Establish intravenous/intraosseous access Take bloods (full blood count, urea and electrolytes) Take blood cultures Take capillary blood gas	*Nurse assistant can ask what the candidate wants them to take via the cannula*	1 1 1 1
Immediate antibiotics		1
Fluid challenge 20 mL/kg	*Nurse assistant can ask if we are going to do anything about the BP*	1

Further developments
The examiner may report that the child remains hypotensive, with BP 60 mmHg, and tachycardic, despite having had three fluid challenges. He is increasingly drowsy.

What additional steps would you like to take?

The manikin vital signs can be set to reflect this change.

Action	Simulation action/response	Marking
This child now needs intubation.		1
Get appropriate help		1
Check airway equipment available: • Bag valve mask and appropriate size ETT • ETT one half-size above/below • Monitoring, including capnography	*Nurse assistant asks what size tube? (age/4 + 4)*	1 1 1
Drugs – any reasonable choice can be justified. Ketamine as an induction agent (1–2 mg/kg) would be a good choice in the presence of shock.	*Nurse assistant can ask why we are using these particular drugs*	1
Draw up and start inotropes (dopamine) prior to intubation	*Nurse assistant can ask if we want to prepare anything else?*	1

Resuscitation 9

Overview

A 60-year-old man develops a blocked tracheostomy which cannot be easily addressed. The tube needs to be removed, which is a big call in a recent percutaneous tracheostomy, but the airway can be managed orally.

Key learning objectives/assessment criteria

- Manage obstructed tracheostomy in potentially patent upper airway
- Describe the pros and cons of a double cannula tube

Background for candidates

You are on the intensive care unit and are called to see a 60-year-old man who has been on the unit for 2 weeks and is recovering from an infective exacerbation of chronic obstructive pulmonary disease (COPD). He required mechanical ventilation for 10 days and, after a failed extubation, he had a percutaneous tracheostomy performed 2 days ago. He has a single-lumen cuffed tracheostomy *in situ*, which has not been changed. He has been weaning steadily and was breathing spontaneously via a tracheostomy mask and 40% O_2.

His HR is 120 bpm and RR 45 bpm with obvious use of the accessory muscles of respiration. His SpO_2 is 86%. There is no vocalization.

The nurse asks you to see him as he has started to desaturate and is not responding to her.

Information for simulation facilitators

Initial set-up

- Critical care environment
- Obstructed (with tape, blue tac or something similar) single-lumen tracheostomy *in situ*
- Cuff up
- HR 120 bpm, BP 160/100 mmHg
- RR 45 bpm, ventilating spontaneously, SpO_2 88%
- Green National Tracheostomy Safety Project (NTSP) bedhead sign (patent airway – normal upper airway) – see www.tracheostomy.org.uk
- No capnography waveform at outset

  Manikin note: Probably no airflow will be detected at the trachea or mouth (depending on the manikin). If they deflate the cuff at some point, sometimes you will get airflow at the mouth. Make the manikin apnoeic before this point.

You will need:

- Tracheostomy mask
- Spare NRB Mask with green oxygen tubing
- Bougie
- Spare tracheostomy tube

- Intubation equipment including an endotracheal tube (ETT), laryngeal mask airway (LMA) and bougie
- Waters' circuit
- Suction catheters to fit down tracheostomy
- Capnography tubing
- One nurse assistant

Progress and mark scheme

Initial assessment

Expect an ABCDE approach from the candidate.

Action	Simulation action/response	Marking
Decide at outset that this is a tracheostomy patient with a potentially patent upper airway. Follow the patent upper airway algorithm.		1
Call for help (anaesthetics/critical care senior help. Surgeon is useful but not essential)		1
Administer 100% O_2 to the face via a new face-mask		1
AND 100% O_2 to the tracheostomy initially by turning up the FiO_2 of the tracheostomy mask circuit, or by attaching a Waters' circuit		1
Ask for waveform capnography Is the patient breathing spontaneously? Check at face and trachea	*Minimal ventilation. Manikin's chest will move up and down. Bag doesn't move (if Waters' circuit attached and no O_2 supply). No mouth breathing. This should take candidate down the 'obstructed' trachea route. If they are unsure, then stop the manikin breathing – respiratory arrest.*	1 1 1
Check for inner tube – there is no inner tube	*If they ask:* • *Is there any mouth breathing?* '*No*' • *Look for subcutaneous emphysema. None* • *Check for obvious displacement, blood or secretions. Not obviously displaced* • *Exclude a speaking valve. None present* • *Is there an inner tube?* '*No*'	1
Check patency of tracheostomy with suction catheter.	*Suction catheter will not pass*	1
Deflate the trachy tube cuff. Reassess mouth and trachy breathing. No breathing detected at mouth or trachy.	*Need to make manikin apnoeic here*	1 1

Further developments: removal of tracheostomy and emergency oxygenation

The patient continues to deteriorate with SpO$_2$ 75% on 100% O$_2$. Manikin becomes apnoeic and unresponsive. *Make the manikin unable to be ventilated and stop breathing.*

Action	Simulation action/response	Marking
Decide that the tube is blocked or displaced and is hampering ventilation	*There are no spontaneous breaths* *If the candidate doesn't remove the tracheostomy, progress to severe bradycardia (as a hint!) Pause scenario here until they remove the tracheostomy.*	1
Remove the blocked tracheostomy		1
Reassess ventilation via stoma and mouth		1
Cover stoma and ventilate using face-mask (or LMA) Attempt to oxygenate via stoma (LMA or paediatric face-mask) if unsuccessful	*Manikin deteriorates slowly until oral oxygenation is attempted.* *Drop SpO$_2$ if candidate attempts stoma ventilation.* *Unable to insert new trachy tube if attempted*	2
Prepare for oral intubation	*Nurse prompts:*	1
Request uncut ETT	*'What are we going to do now?'*	1
Difficult intubation equipment	*'What do you need'*	1

If the candidate attempts to reinsert a new tracheostomy tube into the stoma, tell them that the stoma has virtually closed and this is impossible. They could argue that a bougie or endoscope could be tried. Oral re-intubation is probably the safest option with a new percutaneous tracheostomy.

Resuscitation 10

Overview

A 30-year-old woman suffers an anaphylactic reaction to an antibiotic on a surgical ward and the candidate is called to assess her. Initial resuscitation does not help and she develops a cardiac arrest.

Key learning objectives/assessment criteria

- Rapid assessment of the patient
- Knowledge of initial treatment of anaphylaxis
- Management of cardiac arrest

Background for candidates

A 30-year-old lady has been admitted to a surgical ward with suspected cholecystitis. Her past medical history is otherwise unremarkable. The junior doctor has just given her a dose of antibiotic and she has become short of breath and feels faint within 10 minutes. The doctor and a nurse have asked for your help as she looks awful and they are really worried that this might be a severe reaction to the antibiotic.

Information for simulation facilitators

Initial set-up

- Manikin laid on bed
- Ward-based – oximeter, non-invasive BP, no ECG
- Wheeze, RR 34 bpm
- HR 140 bpm, BP 65/40
- Capillary refill 6 seconds
- Rash if possible under clothes

You will need:

- Mock induction and vasopressor drugs (including adrenaline)
- Intravenous fluids
- Intravenous access
- Training defibrillator
- Airway management equipment
- One doctor and one nurse for the cardiopulmonary resuscitation (CPR)

Initial vital signs:
- HR 140 bpm sinus
- Non-invasive BP 65/40 mmHg
- RR 34 bpm
- SpO$_2$ 90%

Progress and mark scheme

Action	Simulation action/response	Marking
Check/assess airway	Patient opens eyes to voice, groaning	1
Apply 100% FiO$_2$ via non-rebreather mask		1
Assess breathing: • Inspection, palpation, percussion and auscultation • Check O$_2$ saturation	AE symmetrical with widespread wheeze. O$_2$ saturation not recording	1 1
Assess circulation – HR, BP, capillary refill	BP 65/40 mmHg HR 140 bpm, regular, capillary refill 6 seconds	1
Large-bore intravenous access Blood for full blood count, urea and electrolytes, cross-match Fluid challenge as low BP Arterial blood gas		1 (both) 1 (both)
Assess disability: AVPU or GCS Check blood glucose	Eye opens to voice BM is 4.2	1
Expose patient	Widespread rash	1
Recognize anaphylaxis		1
Drugs: • Adrenaline 0.5 mg (intramuscular) • Chlorphenamine 10 mg (intravenous) • Hydrocortisone 200 mg (intravenous) • Salbutamol nebulizer		1 1 1 1
Patient has cardiac arrest		
Call for help		1
Commence CPR 30:2		1
Attach defibrillation pads and recognize pulseless electrical activity arrest		1
Airway management/ intubation		1

(cont.)

Action	Simulation action/response	Marking
Recognize and treat reversible causes (4 'H's and 4 'T's)	Hypotension, hypoxia, hyper/hypo kalaemia/thermia Toxins, thrombo-embolism, tamponade, tension pneumothorax	1
Intravenous adrenaline 1 mg		1

The cardiac arrest should continue until the candidate has had the chance to comment on the reversible causes of the cardiac arrest and give an adrenaline bolus. In practice settings, the manikin may resume a circulation if time allows and discussion about post arrest care could include the role of adrenaline infusions, mast cell tryptase and airway management in the patient with anaphylaxis (difficult).

Appendix: Curriculum mapping

Section I: Data interpretation

	Title of question	Domain/syllabus map
Data 1	Acid base	2.5, 4.8
Data 2	Methaemoglobin	2.5, 2.6, 3.10, 4.1
Data 3	Infective diarrhoea and toxic megacolon	2.6, 4.1, 11.2, 11.3
Data 4	Major burn	1.6
Data 5	Ruptured hemidiaphragm	2.2, 2.6, 2.8, 5.7
Data 6	Post cardiac arrest	1.3, 3.3, 3.6
Data 7	Necrotizing fasciitis	3.1, 4.2
Data 8	ARDS	2.6, 3.8
Data 9	Stridor	2.6, 3.1
Data 10	Hyponatraemia	3.1, 3.2
Data 11	Chest drain in liver	2.6, 3.3, 11.4
Data 12	Interpretation of pulmonary function tests	2.8
Data 13	Serotonin syndrome	?.8, 3.10
Data 14	Propofol infusion syndrome	2.3, 2.8, 4.1
Data 15	Guillain–Barré Syndrome	2.8, 3.6
Data 16	Epidural management	5.16
Data 17	Panton–Valentine leukocidin (PVL) MRSA pneumonia	2.4, 2.6, 3.8. 3.9, 4.2
Data 18	Surviving (urological) sepsis	2.5, 2.6, 2.7, 3.9
Data 19	Ventilator-associated pneumonia	2.6, 4.2, 11.4, 11.6
Data 20	Refeeding syndrome	4.9
Data 21	Acute coronary syndrome and papillary muscle rupture	2.6, 3.3, 4.5
Data 22	TTP/HUS	2.7, 2.8, 3.4
Data 23	Subarachnoid haemorrhage	2.6, 3.6
Data 24	Post oesophagectomy anastomotic leak	2.6, 5.1, 6.1,
Data 25	Pulmonary embolism	2.3, 2.6, 3.3
Data 26	Heparin-induced thrombocytopenia	2.8, 11.4
Data 27	Brainstem death	2.6, 8.4
Data 28	Tricyclic overdose	2.3, 3.10

(cont.)

	Title of question	Domain/syllabus map
Data 29	Chest-pain assessment	2.1, 2.6
Data 30	Intra-abdominal hypertension	2.6, 2.8, 3.7
Data 31	Selective decontamination of the digestive tract	4.2
Data 32	Bone marrow transplant	2.6, 2.8, 6.4
Data 33	Acute kidney injury	2.8, 3.2, 3.4
Data 34	Broncho-pleural fistula	1.5, 2.6
Data 35	Myasthenia gravis	3.6
Data 36	RV infarct	2.3, 3.3, 4.4
Data 37	Rhabdomyolysis	2.3, 4.7, 4.8
Data 38	Cerebrovascular accident	2.6, 3.6, 6.3
Data 39	Acute leukaemia	2.8, 3.1
Data 40	Diabetic ketoacidosis	2.8, 4.8
Data 41	Failure to wean	7.1
Data 42	Pleural effusion	2.6, 2.8
Data 43	Intensive care unit follow-up clinic anaemia	2.2, 2.8
Data 44	Acute liver failure	2.6, 2.8, 3.5
Data 45	Cirrhosis with upper gastro-intestinal bleeding	3.5, 5.18
Data 46	Sedation and sedation scoring	7.3
Data 47	Encephalitis, epilepsy and MRI scans	2.6, 3.6
Data 48	Acute renal failure in an HIV-positive man	1.4, 3.1, 3.4, 4.2,
Data 49	Digoxin toxicity and cardiac pacing	2.3, 2.8, 3.10, 5.12
Data 50	Acute pancreatitis.	2.6, 2.8, 3.7, 11.7
Data 51	Cortisol and thyroxine in the critically ill	2.8, 3.1
Data 52	TEG and major haemorrhage	2.8, 3.3
Data 53	Poisoning	3.10
Data 54	Electrocardiogram interpretation	2.3
Data 55	Chest X-ray interpretation	2.6

Section II: Equipment

	Title of question	Domain/syllabus map
Equipment 1	Arterial lines	5.8
Equipment 2	Tracheostomy weaning and communication	4.6, 5.6
Equipment 3	Bronchoscopy	5.5
Equipment 4	Cooling devices	1.3
Equipment 5	Pulmonary artery catheter	5.14
Equipment 6	Nasogastric tubes	5.19
Equipment 7	High-flow nasal cannula	5.1
Equipment 8	Cardiac output technologies	5.14
Equipment 9	Catheter-related bloodstream infection and vancomycin-resistant enterococcus	4.2, 11.4, 11.6
Equipment 10	Spinal needles	5.15
Equipment 11	Capnography	2.7
Equipment 12	Patient transfer	10.1
Equipment 13	Tracheostomies	5.6
Equipment 14	Central lines	5.9, 5.10
Equipment 15	Haemofiltration	4.7
Equipment 16	Intra-aortic balloon pump	3.3, 4.5

Section III: Ethics and communication

	Title of question	Domain/syllabus map
Ethics 1	Anaphylaxis	12.1
Ethics 2	Pulmonary embolism	12.1
Ethics 3	Malignant hyperthermia	3.1, 12.1
Ethics 4	Organ donation	8.2, 12.1, 12.4
Ethics 5	End-of-life care	8.2, 12.1, 12.4, 12.12
Ethics 6	Muscular dystrophy	3.2, 12.1, 12.4, 12.12
Ethics 7	Delirium	7.2
Ethics 8	Deterioration post discharge	12.1, 12.2, 12.7, 12.12
Ethics 9	Consent for tracheostomy	12.1, 12.4, 12.12
Ethics 10	Blood transfusion	4.3
Ethics 11	Alcoholic liver disease	2.2, 2.4, 2.8, 12.12
Ethics 12	Long QT	2.3, 3.1, 12.1

Section IV: Resuscitation and simulation

	Title of question	Domain/Syllabus map
Resuscitation 1	Displaced airway	5.1, 5.2, 5.3, 11.4
Resuscitation 2	Child submersion	1.2, 9.1, 9.2
Resuscitation 3	Child with seizures	3.6, 9.1
Resuscitation 4	Bleeding trauma with head injury	1.5
Resuscitation 5	Asthma	1.1, 2.5, 3.1, 5.1, 5.2
Resuscitation 6	Pregnancy and VF arrest	1.2, 3.11, 5.11
Resuscitation 7	Chest opening on the intensive care unit	3.3, 4.4, 6.2
Resuscitation 8	Paediatric sepsis	3.3, 9.1
Resuscitation 9	Tracheostomy emergency	5.1, 5.2, 5.3
Resuscitation 10	Anaphylaxis	1.2, 3.1, 3.3

Index